Brain Development in *Drosophila melanogaster*

ADVANCES IN EXPERIMENTAL MEDICINE AND BIOLOGY

A Continuation Order Plan is available for this series. A continuation order will bring delivery of each new volume immediately upon publication. Volumes are billed only upon actual shipment. For further information please contact the publisher.

Brain Development
in *Drosophila melanogaster*

Edited by

Gerhard M. Technau, PhD

Institute of Genetics, University of Mainz, Mainz, Germany

Springer Science+Business Media, LLC
Landes Bioscience

Springer Science+Business Media, LLC
Landes Bioscience

Printed in the USA

Springer Science+Business Media, LLC, 233 Spring Street, New York, New York 10013, USA
http://www.springer.com

Please address all inquiries to the publishers:
Landes Bioscience, 1002 West Avenue, 2nd Floor, Austin, Texas 78701, USA
Phone: 512/ 637 5060; FAX: 512/ 637 6079
http://www.landesbioscience.com

Brain Development in Drosophila melanogaster, edited by Gerhard M. Technau, Landes Bioscience/
Springer Science+Business Media, LLC dual imprint / Springer series: Advances in Experimental
Medicine and Biology.

ISBN: 978-0-387-78260-7

Library of Congress Cataloging-in-Publication Data

Brain development in Drosophila melanogaster / edited by Gerhard M. Technau.
     p. ; cm.
  Includes bibliographical references.
  ISBN 978-0-387-78260-7
  1. Drosophila melanogaster--Development. 2. Brain--Growth. 3. Developmental neurobiology. I.
Technau, Gerhard M.
  [DNLM: 1. Brain--embryology. 2. Drosophila melanogaster--growth & development. QX 505
B814 2008]
  QL537.D76B73 2008
  595.77'4--dc22
                    2008003551

PREFACE

The central nervous system (CNS) represents the organ with the highest structural and functional complexity. Accordingly, uncovering the mechanisms leading to cell diversity, patterning and connectivity in the CNS is one of the major challenges in developmental biology. The developing CNS of the fruitfly *Drosophila melanogaster* is an ideal model system to study these processes. Several principle questions regarding neurogenesis (like stem cell formation, cell fate specification, axonal pathfinding) have been addressed in *Drosophila* by focusing on the relatively simply structured truncal parts of the nervous system. However, information processing (e.g., vision, olfaction), behavior, learning and memory require highly specialized structures, which are located in the brain. Owing to much higher complexity and hidden segmental organisation, our understanding of brain development is still quite rudimentary. Considerable advances have been made recently in bringing the resolution of brain structures to the level of individual cells and their lineages, which significantly facilitates investigations into the mechanisms controlling brain development.

This book provides an overview of some major facets of recent research on *Drosophila* brain development. The individual chapters were written by experts in each field. V. Hartenstein et al survey the generic cell types that make up the developing brain and describe the morphogenesis of neural lineages and their relationship to neuropil compartments in the larval brain. Recent findings on anteroposterior regionalization and on dorsoventral patterning in the embryonic brain are reviewed in the chapters by R. Lichtneckert and H. Reichert and by R. Urbach and G. Technau, respectively. Both processes show striking parallels between *Drosophila* and mouse. Photoactivated gene expression as a means for tracing cell fate through embryonic brain development is demonstrated in J. Minden's chapter. At present, the best characterized neural network on the developmental, structural, and functional level is the chemosensory system, to which three chapters are devoted: R. Stocker's chapter covers the design of the larval chemosensory system and shows that it prefigures the adult system. V. Rodrigues and T. Hummel summarize recent findings on the specification and connectivity development of the adult olfactory receptor neurons. P. Laissue and B. Vosshall review the molecular biology, neuroanatomy and function of the adult olfactory system. A further focus of research is the visual system, with the optic lobes comprising about half of the adult fly brain. The genetic and cellular principles which direct the assembly of the optic lobes are highlighted in the chapter by K. Fischbach and P. Hiesinger. The central brain harbors distinct neuropils like the central complex and the mushroom bodies, as well as "diffused neuropils" which lack clearly demarcated structures. K. Ito and T. Awasaki review the organization of the adult central brain and show how its complex architecture evolves from clonally related neural circuits.

This book will be helpful to those who want to study brain development in the fly. As knowledge extracted from the *Drosophila* model has often proven to be of more general relevance, comparative aspects are included in most chapters. Therefore, this book should also be useful for researchers working on brain development in other organisms and on brain evolution, as well as for instructors and advanced students in the field of developmental neurobiology.

I would like to thank the authors for producing an excellent series of thoughtful reviews, Ronald Landes for encouraging me to edit this volume, and Cynthia Conomos for continuous support.

Gerhard M. Technau, PhD

ABOUT THE EDITOR...

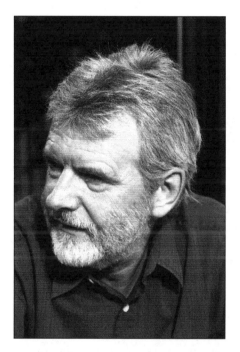

GERHARD M. TECHNAU, PhD, is Professor and Head of the Institute of Genetics at the University of Mainz, Germany. His main research interests include mechanisms controlling the generation of cell diversity and segmental pattern in the nervous system using *Drosophila* as a model. He received his PhD from Würzburg University, and the venia legendi from Cologne University. Awarded a Heisenberg-Fellowship from the Deutsche Forschungsgemeinschaft, he worked at Cologne University and University of California (UCSF) before being recruited by the University of Mainz.

PARTICIPANTS

Takeshi Awasaki
Institute of Molecular
   and Cellular Biosciences
The University of Tokyo
Yayoi, Bunkyo-ku
Tokyo
Japan
and
Department of Neurobiology
University of Massachusetts Medical
   School
Worcester, Massachusetts
USA

Karl-Friedrich Fischbach
Department of Neurobiology
Albert-Ludwigs University
   of Freiburg
Freiburg
Germany

Siaumin Fung
Department of Molecular, Cell
   and Developmental Biology
University of California, Los Angeles
Los Angeles, California
USA

Volker Hartenstein
Department of Molecular, Cell
   and Developmental Biology
University of California, Los Angeles
Los Angeles, California
USA

Peter Robin Hiesinger
Department of Physiology
and
Green Center Division
   for Systems Biology
UT Southwestern Medical Center
Dallas, Texas
USA

Thomas Hummel
Institut füer Neurobiologie
Universitaet Muenster
Muenster
Germany

Kei Ito
Institute of Molecular
   and Cellular Biosciences
The University of Tokyo
Yayoi, Bunkyo-ku
Tokyo
Japan

Philippe P. Laissue
Kent Institute of Medicine
   and Health Sciences
Medical Image Computing
University of Kent
Canterbury, Kent
UK

Robert Lichtneckert
Biozentrum
University of Basel
Basel
Switzerland

Jonathan Minden
Department of Biological Sciences
    and Science
Carnegie Mellon University
Pittsburgh, Pennsylvania
USA

Wayne Pereanu
Department of Molecular, Cell
    and Developmental Biology
University of California, Los Angeles
Los Angeles, California
USA

Heinrich Reichert
Biozentrum
University of Basel
Basel
Switzerland

Veronica Rodrigues
National Centre for Biological
    Sciences
Tata Institute of Fundamental
    Research
Bangalore
India

Shana Spindler
Department of Molecular, Cell
    and Developmental Biology
University of California, Los Angeles
Los Angeles, California
USA

Reinhard F. Stocker
Department of Biology
University of Fribourg
Fribourg
Switzerland

Gerhard M. Technau
Institute of Genetics
University of Mainz
Mainz
Germany

Rolf Urbach
Institute of Genetics
University of Mainz
Mainz
Germany

Leslie B. Vosshall
Laboratory of Neurogenetics
    and Behavior
The Rockefeller University
New York, New York
USA

CONTENTS

4. DISSECTION OF THE EMBRYONIC BRAIN USING PHOTOACTIVATED GENE EXPRESSION 57

Jonathan Minden

5. DESIGN OF THE LARVAL CHEMOSENSORY SYSTEM 69

Reinhard F. Stocker

6. DEVELOPMENT OF THE *DROSOPHILA* OLFACTORY SYSTEM 82

Veronica Rodrigues and Thomas Hummel

7. THE OLFACTORY SENSORY MAP IN *DROSOPHILA*......................... 102

Philippe P. Laissue and Leslie B. Vosshall

8. OPTIC LOBE DEVELOPMENT 115

Karl-Friedrich Fischbach and Peter Robin Hiesinger

9. CLONAL UNIT ARCHITECTURE OF THE ADULT FLY BRAIN....... 137

Kei Ito and Takeshi Awasaki

CHAPTER 1

The Development of the *Drosophila* Larval Brain

Volker Hartenstein,* Shana Spindler, Wayne Pereanu and Siaumin Fung

Abstract

In this chapter we will start out by describing in more detail the progenitors of the nervous system, the neuroblasts and ganglion mother cells. Subsequently we will survey the generic cell types that make up the developing Drosophila brain, namely neurons, glial cells and tracheal cells. Finally, we will attempt a synopsis of the neuronal connectivity of the larval brain that can be deduced from the analysis of neural lineages and their relationship to neuropile compartments.

Synopsis of the Phases and Elements of *Drosophila* Brain Development

The *Drosophila* brain is shaped during three developmental phases that include the embryonic, larval and pupal phase. In the early embryo, a population of neuroblasts (primary neuroblasts; Fig. 1A, top) delaminates from the neurectoderm and generates, in a stem cell-like manner, the glia and neurons that differentiate into the fully functional larval brain (primary neurons and glia). Each neuroblast produces a highly invariant lineage of cells that, at least temporarily, stay together and extend processes that fasciculate into a common bundle (primary axon tract; Fig. 1B). After a phase of mitotic dormancy that lasts from late embryogenesis to the end of the 1st larval instar, the same neuroblasts that had proliferated to form primary neurons during the embryonic period become active again and produce a stereotyped set of secondary lineages (Fig. 1A, center). Neurons of the secondary lineages are delayed in regard to morphological and functional differentiation. They form short, unbranched axons that fasciculate in secondary axon tracts (Fig. 1C). During the pupal phase (metamorphosis) secondary neurons mature and, together with restructured primary neurons, form the adult brain (Fig. 1A, bottom).

The mature *Drosophila* brain of the larva and adult is of the ganglionic type (Fig. 1B, C). Cell bodies of neurons and glial cells form an outer layer, or cortex, around an inner neuropile that consists of highly branched axons and dendrites, as well as synapses formed in between these processes. Because the neuropile is virtually free of cell bodies, it is extraordinarily compact. The typical insect neuron has a neurite that projects throughout a large part of the neuropile (Fig. 1B; see also section 'The Generic Cell Types of the *Drosophila* Brain' below). Tufts of terminal arbors (dendritic and axonal) branch off the neurite close to the cell body (proximal branches) and at its tip (terminal branches; Fig. 1B). Dendritic and axonal branches are assembled into neuropile compartments. Long axons are bundled into tracts that interconnect these compartments (Fig. 1B, C). Glial sheaths envelop the cortex surface (surface glia), groups of neuronal cell bodies (cortex glia) and the neuropile (neuropile glia). Neuropile glial cells also form septa that subdivide the neuropile into several distinct compartments.

*Corresponding Author: Volker Hartenstein—Department of Molecular Cell and Developmental Biology, University of California Los Angeles, Los Angeles, California 90095, USA. Email: volkerh@mcdb.ucla.edu

Brain Development in Drosophila melanogaster, edited by Gerhard M. Technau.
©2008 Landes Bioscience and Springer Science+Business Media.

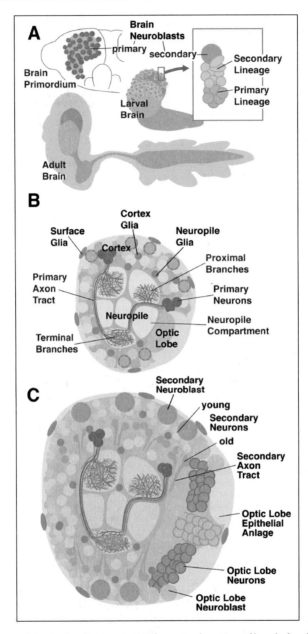

Figure 1. *Drosophila* brain development. A) Schematic drawings of head of early embryo (top), larval brain (center left), neuroblast lineage (center right) and adult brain (bottom). Primary brain neuroblasts (dark lilac) delaminate from the head neurectoderm and produce primary lineages that form the larval brain (light lilac). In the late larva neuroblasts start producing secondary lineages (orange) that are integrated with the primary neurons into the adult brain. (B, C) Schematic cross sections of one brain hemisphere of early larva (B) and late larva (C). Primary neuroblasts and neurons are shaded lilac; secondary neuroblasts and neurons are in orange. Two clusters of primary neurons are highlighted to show projection of neurites. Glia cells are colored green.

In this chapter we will start out by describing in more detail the progenitors of the nervous system, the neuroblasts and ganglion mother cells. Subsequently we will survey the generic cell types that make up the developing *Drosophila* brain, namely neurons, glial cells and tracheal cells. Finally, we will attempt a synopsis of the neuronal connectivity of the larval brain that can be deduced from the analysis of neural lineages and their relationship to neuropile compartments.

Progenitors of the *Drosophila* Brain: Neuroblasts and Ganglion Mother Cells

The Primary Phase of Neuroblast Activity in the Embryo

The brain of insects and some other arthropod taxa is formed by a unique type of stem cell-like progenitor cell called a neuroblast. Neural progenitors of this type are not found in vertebrates or (as far as known to date) other invertebrate phyla. Neuroblasts delaminate from the embryonic neurectoderm and form a cell layer sandwiched in between the ectoderm and mesoderm (Fig. 2A). The pattern of neuroblasts is invariant. Thus, each neuroblast forms a uniquely identifiable cell that appears at the same time and position in every individual of a given species. Neuroblast patterns are very similar even when comparing different insect species such as *Drosophila* and grasshopper. Neuroblasts appear in two broad regions of the embryo. The head (procephalic) neurectoderm, located in the anterior-dorsal part of the ectoderm, gives rise to neuroblasts that form the brain (Fig. 2B). The ventral neurectoderm, stretching out along the trunk ectoderm, produces the neuroblasts of the ventral nerve cord. Neuroblasts are organized segmentally, with each segment giving rise to an identical segmental set, called neuromere, of approximately 25 neuroblasts per side. The brain, a composite structure formed by the fusion of several modified neuromeres, contains approximately 100 neuroblasts per side.[1,2]

After delamination from the ectoderm, neuroblasts form a layer of large, rounded cells inside the embryo. Soon these cells proliferate in what is known as a stem cell mode (Fig. 2C). Thus, whereas most cells in an embryo divide symmetrical, with both daughter cells being of about the same size and fate, neuroblasts divide asymmetrically into one large and one small daughter cell with very different fates. The large cell (still called a neuroblast) continues dividing in the stem cell mode for a variable number of rounds of divisions. Most primary neuroblasts in the embryo divide 5-8 times, with a cell cycle duration of 45-60min;[3] secondary neuroblasts may divide 50 times or more (V.H., unpublished). The small cell resulting from a neuroblast mitosis, called a ganglion mother cell (GMC), typically divides only one more time 60-90min after its birth.[3] The two daughter cells of the GMC become postmitotic and differentiate into neurons or glial cells. Since the mitotic spindle of neuroblasts is typically directed perpendicular to the plane of the neuroblast layer, ganglion mother cells and immature neurons form a stack on top of the neuroblast from which they originated (Fig. 2A,C). In this manner, all cells of a neuroblast lineage remain spatially close to each other and are arranged along a spatio-temporal gradient. Neuroblasts and ganglion mother cells are situated externally at the brain surface (Fig. 2D,G), adjacent to the last born (youngest) neurons. Early born (old) neurons are the most remote from the neuroblast, bordering the nascent neuropile. The layered organization of the brain cortex can be analyzed in detail by using molecular markers that are expressed at different stages of neuroblast proliferation and neuronal differentiation (Fig. 2G,H).[4]

Secondary Neuroblasts and GMCs of the Larval Brain

The last rounds of primary neuroblast division occur at embryonic stages 14-15 (Fig. 2E); after that stage, only GMC divisions are recognizable for another 2-3 hours (Fig. 2F). Neuroblasts become mitotically inactive and shrink in size, so that they cannot be recognized in first instar brains (Fig. 3A). A small set of neuroblasts, including the four mushroom body neuroblasts and one of the basal anterior neuroblasts (for classification of neuroblasts and their lineages, see section 'Neuroanatomy of the Developing *Drosophila* Brain' of this chapter), escape the general arrest of neuroblast activity and continue to proliferate throughout the early larval period (Fig. 3A,B).[5]

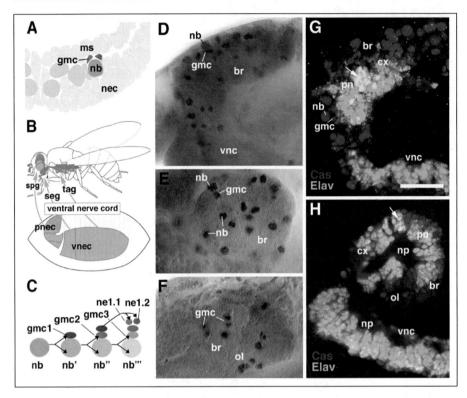

Figure 2. Primary neuroblasts and ganglion mother cells. A) Schematic cross section of early embryo showing ventral neurectoderm (nec), mesoderm (ms), neuroblast layer (nb) and ganglion mother cells (gmc). B) Schematic of blastoderm fate map (bottom) and adult fly CNS (top). Anlage of ventral neurectoderm (vnec) gives rise to ventral nerve cord which becomes the thoraco-abdominal ganglion (tag) and subesophageal ganglion (seg) of the adult brain. Procephalic neurectoderm (pnec) gives rise to the supraesophageal ganglion (spg) of the adult brain. C) Asymmetric division of neuroblast (nb) into second order neuroblasts (nb', nb''....) and ganglion mother cells (gmc,1 gmc2....). Ganglion mother cells divide one time equally into two neurons (ne1.1, ne1.2). D-F) Lateral views of embryonic brain (br) and ventral nerve cord (vnc) at stage 12 (D), stage 15 (E) and stage 16 (F). Mitotic neuroblasts (nb) and ganglion mother cells (gmc) are labeled with antiPhosphohistone (a marker for mitosis). The proliferating cells form a dense layer at the outer surface of the brain (D). The last primary neuroblast divisions take place during stage 15 (E); at stage 16, only scattered divisions of GMCs and optic lobe progenitors (ol) occur. G, H) Lateral views of embryonic brain at stage 12 (G) and 16 (H). The transcriptional regulator Castor (Cas; red) is switched on at the stage when neuroblasts undergo their third or fourth division.[4] From that stage onward, Cas is expressed continuously in primary neuroblasts and, transiently, in their progeny. Double-label experiments using Cas and Elav (green) as markers visualize an inner cortex of Elav-positive, postmitotic neurons, an outer layer of Cas-positive neuroblasts and GMCs and an intermediate layer of late born neurons that are already positive for Elav and still express Cas. Other abbreviations: cx, cortex; np, neuropile; pn, primary neurons. Bar: 20 μm.

During the roughly one day period encompassing the second larval instar, the remainder of the neuroblasts are also reactivated (in a pattern that has not yet been studied in detail), so that during the entire third instar the entire complement of neuroblasts is proliferating.

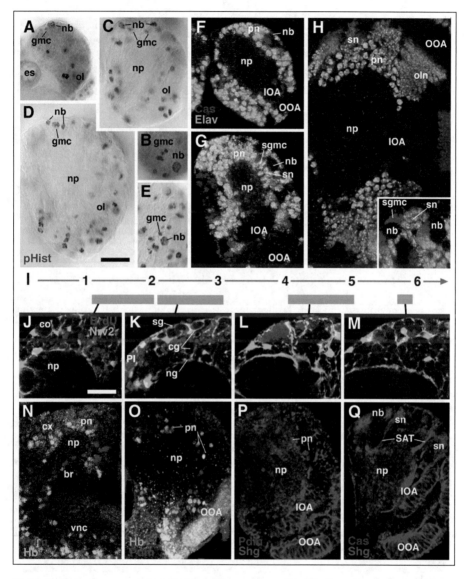

Figure 3. Secondary neuroblasts and ganglion mother cells of the larval brain. A-E) Posterior view of larval brains (A,B) 24 h after egg laying (AEL), first instar; C) 48 h AEL, second instar; (D, E) 72 h AEL, early third instar) labeled with antiPhosphohistone. In early larva (A, B) neuroblasts (nb) and GMCs of mushroom body are labeled; proliferation is also detected in the primordium of the optic lobe (ol). More neuroblasts begin secondary phase of proliferation during the second instar (C); during early third instar (D, E), all neuroblasts are active. (F-H: Confocal sections of larval brains 48 h AEL (F), 72 h AEL (G) and 120h AEL (H; inset in H shows secondary lineages at higher magnification). Labeling of neurons with anti-Elav (green) and neuroblasts, GMCs and young secondary neurons (sn) with antiCas (red). Cas is expressed transiently in secondary neuroblasts when they reactivate (F); at later stages, Cas is found in GMCs and newly born secondary neurons (G, H; inset in H). Note size difference between primary neurons (pn in H) and secondary neurons. Legend continued on following page.

Figure 3, continued from previous page. I-M: BrdU pulse chase experiments visualizing the correlation between birth date and neuron location. J-M show confocal cross sections of dorsal brain hemisphere of 3rd instar larva. Glia cells (labeled green by Nrv2-Gal4 driving UAS-GFP) outline the brain surface (sg surface glia), the cortex (cg cortex glia; co cortex) and the neuropile surface (ng neuropile glia; np neuropile). Larvae were fed with BrdU during time intervals indicated by gray bars in time line (panel I; numbers indicate days after fertilization). The location of BrdU labeled neurons (red in J-M) within the cortex correlates with the time of BrdU incorporation: early born neurons occupy a deep location in the cortex, late born neurons are superficial. N) Confocal section of late embryonic brain showing expression of the transcription factors Hunchback (Hb; green) and Pdm (red) in primary neurons (pn) born during the first and third round of division of neuroblasts. O) Confocal section of early third instar larval brain. Hb and Pdm are not reactivated in secondary neuroblasts, but stay expressed in primary neurons (presumably the same that had turned on expression in the early embryo) located in the deep cortex. P, Q) Confocal section of early third instar larval brain. Secondary lineages (sn), glia and optic lobe (IOA: inner optic anlage; OOA outer optic anlage) are labeled with antiShg (DEcadherin) antibody (blue). Cas expression (red in Q) overlaps with secondary lineages; Pdm (red in P) is restricted to primary neurons near neuropile. Other abbreviations: br, brain; es, esophagus; np, neuropile; oln, optic lobe neurons; sgmc, secondary GMC; PI, pars intercerebralis; SAT, secondary axon tract; vnc, ventral nerve cord Bar: 20 μm

Labeling of neuroblasts and GMCs of the larva reveals that these cells, just like their embryonic counterparts, are located at the brain surface (Fig. 3A-E).[6-8] The orientation of the mitotic spindle in secondary neuroblasts appears to be much more variable than in primary neuroblasts, ranging from parallel to perpendicular relative to the brain surface.[6,9] This could in part be due to the fact that the mechanism controlling spindle orientation could be quite different: in the embryo, neuroblasts are in contact with the epithelial neurectoderm and "inherit" from the neurectoderm a protein complex, the Inscuteable complex, that remains apical and plays a role in tethering the mitotic spindle to the membrane in such a way that results in a vertical orientation.[10-12] Secondary neuroblasts in the larva have no contact with the ectoderm (or epidermis); rather, they are surrounded on all sides by a glial layer (see below). Thus, the mechanism that controls the mitotic spindle orientation, as well as the onset and frequency of mitosis, is likely to be controlled by glia-neuroblast interactions.[7,13] Within the secondary neuroblast, protein complexes orienting the spindle appear to be the same as in the embryo. Thus, members of the Par complex, including Baz, Par,6 and aPKC, localize to an apical crescent along with Inscuteable, while Miranda and Prospero localize to the basal crescent (Fig. 4E).[6,9]

Despite the variability of neuroblast mitotic spindle orientation, the larval brain cortex is organized into concentric layers where the location of a neuron reflects its birth date. This correlation between birth date and location of a neuron can be visualized by pulse chase experiments in which BrdU is fed to larvae at different time intervals (Fig. 3I-M), or with the expression of molecular markers such as Cas, Pdm or Hb (Fig. 3F-H, N-Q).[14] Primary neurons are the deepest cells (Fig. 3H, O, P), bordering the neuropile; late born secondary neurons are superficial, surrounding the neuroblasts (Fig. 3H, M, Q).

Control of Drosophila *Neuroblast Proliferation*

As described in the previous section, the *Drosophila* brain undergoes two periods of growth through the activation and quiescence of larval neuroblasts. Interestingly, not all neuroblasts are active at a given time and many sustain extended periods of quiescence before larval division. The molecular factors that control the length of neuroblast quiescence; re-entrance into the S phase of division; the amount of division to occur; and the life-span of the neuroblast are all important issues that must be addressed in order to understand brain growth. In recent studies, light has been shed on a few key molecular pathways that appear to influence neuroblast activities (reviewed in[13,15,16]). Both negative and positive regulators of proliferation cooperate to ensure the proper expansion of the central nervous system as the larva enters puparium formation and eventually adulthood (Fig. 4E).

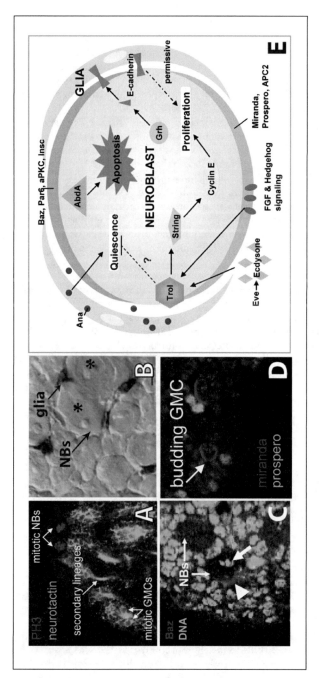

Figure 4. Mechanism of Neuroblast Proliferation. A) Mitotic neuroblasts divide to self-renew and produce a daughter ganglion mother cell, which subsequently divides into two neurons. Mitotic neuroblasts and GMCs (red), neuroblast progeny (green). B) Second instar larval brain expressing the *anachronism* (ana)-lacZ marker. Ana is only expressed by glia (brown stain) and not by the neuroblasts (marked with asterisk). [from Ebens et al Cell, Vol. 74, 15-27, with permission]. C) Bazooka (Baz), a member of the Par-complex, localizes to only the apical crescent of a metaphase neuroblast in this third instar brain. Baz antibody (red, arrowhead); DNA labeled with sytox green (green, arrow). D) Miranda and Prospero are segregated to the basal neuroblast and eventually the budding GMC (arrow). Miranda (red); Prospero (green). E) Molecular pathways involved in the control of brain neuroblast proliferation. The neuroblast is found in three states: quiescence, proliferation, or undergoing apoptosis. Ana allows for a quiescent state, while many pathways act through Trol to initiate proliferation. In addition, the presence of DE-cadherin appears to be a permissive factor in proliferation. During mitosis, a number of factors (e.g., members of the Par complex) localize to the apical cortex of the neuroblast, while other factors (Miranda, Prospero and APC2) localize to a basal crescent and are eventually segregated into the budding GMC. Lastly, in some neuroblasts factors such as the homeobox gene AbdA induce apoptosis to limit the number of mitotic divisions.

Among the negative regulators of neuroblast proliferation are the Hox genes and Anachronism (Ana), a glycoprotein that is secreted from a subpopulation of surface glial cells and is required for retaining neuroblasts in the G1 phase of the cell cycle. In ana mutant larvae, both the optic lobe and central brain neuroblasts begin proliferation prematurely.[17] Because Ana originates in adjacent glial cells, the idea that glial cells act similar to a stem-cell "niche" by mediating neuroblast re-entrance into the cell cycle is tempting. While Ana temporarily delays the onset of division, the posterior Hox genes restrict neuroblast proliferation by inducing apoptosis in neuroblasts.[18] Thus, once neuroblasts of the abdominal neuromeres (and, by inference, other neuroblasts as well) have reached the correct number of cell divisions, a pulse of AbdA expression initiates programmed cell death, thereby delimiting the number of neuroblast divisions.

A key player in the mechanism that initiates neuroblast division is Trol, the *Drosophila* homologue of mammalian Perlecan, a large multidomain heparan sulfate proteoglycan residing in the ECM.[19] Like mammalian Perlecan, *Drosophila* Trol has been shown to mediate signals through the FGF and Hedgehog pathways.[20] In the larval central nervous system, Trol is required for neuroblast re-entrance into S-phase. Cell division maintenance, however, does not appear to be influenced by Trol expression. Epistasis experiments initially suggested that Trol acts downstream of Ana, by inhibiting Ana or members of an Ana pathway in the quiescent neuroblast.[21] Later studies found, however, that induction of Cyclin E rescues the *trol* mutant phenotype, but does not phenocopy ana mutants.[22,23] Therefore, it is likely another mechanism exists, alone or in conjunction with the Trol pathway, to act as a negative regulator of ana-mediated repression of neuroblast division (Fig. 4).

Given the importance of cell-cell interactions in regulating neuroblast proliferation it comes as no surprise that adhesion molecules and the molecular networks they form part of play a role (Fig. 4). *Drosophila* E-cadherin (DEcad) has a widespread expression in neuroblasts, secondary neurons and glial cells and expression of a dominant negative DE-cadherin leads to reduced neuronal proliferation, resulting in the absence of neurons and axon tracts.[7,8] Because this effect can be phenocopied by expressing the dominant-negative construct in glial cells alone, DEcad most likely mediates interactions between neuroblasts and the glial "niche" during neuroblast proliferation.[7] Grainyhead, a transcription factor present in all post-embryonic neuroblasts, has been shown to directly increase DEcad expression in proliferating neuroblasts.[24] APC1 and APC2, a pair of cytoplasmic proteins that bind to the cadherin-catenin complex and play a role in the context of Wg/Wnt signaling, have been found to be involved in *Drosophila* neuroblast proliferation as well.[25]

The Generic Cell Types of the *Drosophila* Brain

Neurons

The use of molecular markers or DiI injections reveals that the large majority of *Drosophila* larval brain neurons conform to the prototypical architecture which is typical for insect neurons (Fig. 5A).[26] Neurons are unipolar and project their single axon centripetally towards the neuropile. At or near the point where it crosses the boundary between cortex and neuropile, the neurite gives off a collateral that forms a tuft of higher order branches (proximal branches). After continuing for various distances within the neuropile, the neurite ends in a tuft of terminal branches. The neurite can be bifurcated or trifurcated, in which case it produces multiple tufts of terminal branches. In many cases where entire lineages of neurons were labeled, neurites of neurons of a given lineage behave alike, traveling together in a cohesive axon bundle (the primary or secondary axon tract) and branching in the same or closely adjacent neuropile compartments.

The intrinsic neurons of the mushroom body (Kenyon cells) are a good example to illustrate these principles (Fig. 5B).[27-30] Initially, these cells, formed by four contiguous neuroblasts, send their axons in a tight bundle straight anteriorly. Subsequently, proximal (dendritic) branches form near the cell body. The distal tip of Kenyon cell axons trifurcate, forming the dorsal lobe, medial lobe and the spur. Larval Kenyon cells also exemplify the more general point (how general it is remains to be seen through future anatomical studies) that neurons belonging to one lineage have a similar

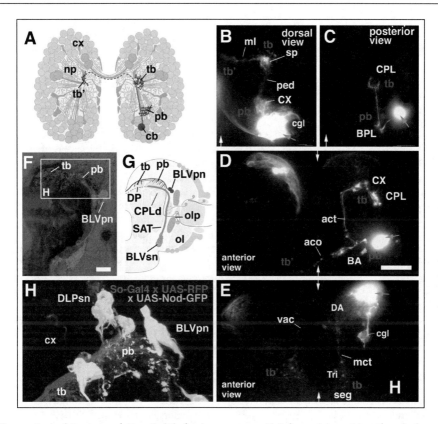

Figure 5. Architecture of *Drosophila* brain neurons. A) Schematic section of early larval brain (cx cortex; np neuropile. One neuron is highlighted in red (cb cell body; pb proximal branches; tb and tb' terminal branches. B-E: Photographs of early larval brain primary neurons injected with DiI (white; blue arrows indicate injection sites; white arrows show midline). B) Kenyon cell of mushroom body (MB). cx calyx; ml medial lobe; ped peduncle; sp spur. C) DPL-type neuron located in postero-lateral cortex. The example shown forms short proximal branches in the BPL compartment and projects a single neurite with terminal branches in the CPL compartment. D) baso-anterior (BA) neuron with proximal dendritic tuft innervating the neuropile of the antennal lobe (BA compartment); the neurite then bifurcates and sends one branch across the antennal commissure (aco) to the contralateral antennal lobe and one branch through the antenno-cerebral tract (act) towards the calyx (CX) and CPL compartment. E) dorso-anterior-medial (DAM) neuron, forming short proximal branches in the ipsilateral dorso-anterior (DA) compartment, close to the location of the cell body; the neurite bifurcates and one branch continues ventrally towards the ipsilateral tritocerebral (Tri) and subesophageal neuropile; the second branch crosses the midline in the ventro-anterior commissure (vac) and descends towards the contralateral tritocerebrum/subesophageal neuropile. F, G) Z-projection of confocal sections (F) and schematic drawing (G) of third instar larval brain showing Sine oculis (So) primary neurons (BLVpn) and secondary neurons (BLVsn; red). The BLVpn has proximal brances (pb) in the CPLd compartment and a set of terminal branches (tb) in the more medially located DP compartment; the axon continues across the midline to form a second set of terminal branches in the contralteral hemisphere (not shown). H) expression of GFP in entire Sine oculis (So)-positive lineage (red) and of the dendritic marker Nod (green) in proximal branches, supporting the idea that these branches are dendrites. Other abbreviations: DLPsn) So-positive neurons of the DLP lineage; cgl, cortex glia; mct, medial cervical tract; ol, optic lobe; olp, optic lobe pioneer; SAT, secondary axon tract; seg, subesophageal ganglion Bars: 20 μm

projection pattern. Thus, dendritic branches of Kenyon cells remain in close contact and, together with axonal trees of afferent fibers (mainly derived from the antennal lobe), form a compact neuropile compartment, called the calyx. Tightly packed axonal branches of Kenyon cells, along with the dendritic trees of postsynaptic cells,[31] give rise to the peduncle, lobe compartments and spur of the mushroom body. Figure 5C–E show three additional examples of DiI filled neurons whose branching pattern conforms to the same prototype. Preliminary data show that many secondary lineages that differentiate during the pupal period conform to the mushroom body lineages with regard to their proximal branching (V.H. and W.P., unpublished). Thus, proximal arborizations of most (if not all) neurons belonging to a given lineage appear to share in the same compartment. Terminal axonal arborization, on the other hand, are typically more diverse. Previous work on primary lineages of the ventral nerve cord had also shown that (terminal) arborizations in this part of the CNS are also quite diverse within a given lineage.[32,33]

In very few instances, such as the Kenyon cells or some olfactory interneurons, has it actually been shown that proximal branches of central neurons correspond to dendrites.[34,35] Molecular differences between dendrites and axons have been reported that in principle can be used to distinguish between the two. For example, the minus-end directed microtubule binding protein Nod 1 accumulates in the dendrites of bipolar sensory neurons and the mushroom body's Kenyon cells and therefore potentially represents a marker of dendrites in the CNS.[36] As shown in Figure 5, Nod1-GFP driven in a small subset of primary neurons that belong to the sine *oculis* (*so*) expressing BLV1 lineage also accumulates in the subset of neurite branches that are close to the cell bodies, indicating that these branches are dendrites.[37,38]

Figure 6 illustrates how the branching pattern of neurons belonging to a lineage evolves over time. To label lineages, the FLP/FRT technique was used.[28] Each panel shows a member of the DAL lineages, a group of lineages located antero-laterally in the brain (for more detail see section 'Neuroanatomy of the Developing *Drosophila* Brain' of this chapter), at different stages of its development. A lineage at embryonic stage 14 (12-14h; Fig. 5A,A') appears as a cluster of contiguous cell bodies capped by a neuroblast, sending a short, unbranched PAT towards the center of the brain primordium. A late embryonic clone (16h; Fig. 6B,B') still exhibits a compact PAT, but short branches have appeared close to the cell body and, in many cases, at the PAT tip. In the early larva, branching of axons has increased dramatically (Fig. 6C,C'). Furthermore, the close packing of cell bodies and their axons has loosened up, although cells and neurites of one lineage are still close to each other. A similar picture presents itself if clones induced in the embryo are visualized in late larvae. Primary neurons branch over much of the neuropile; in addition, secondary lineages have now been added. Secondary neurons are always externally adjacent to the primary neurons. The secondary axon tract penetrates into the thicket of primary branches, suggesting that interactions between the primary axons and SAT exist. Clones induced in the early larva and visualized in the late larva (Fig. 6E) contain exclusively secondary neurons, demonstrating the immature, unbranched nature of secondary axons. Proximal and terminal branches of secondary neurons are formed starting at 12h of pupal development (Fig. 6G). Most lineages have proximal ("dendritic") branches restricted to one compartment, or part thereof. By contrast, terminal branches are typically more widespread, but can also be fairly restricted, as in the case of the DAL lineage shown whose terminal arbors are restricted to a layer of the ellipsoid body.

Glial Cells

Neurons of the *Drosophila* brain are supported by a complex scaffold of glial cells that is established during late embryonic stages. Insect glial cells fall into three classes,[39-42] each of which is represented in the larval brain (Fig. 7A-F). Surface (subperineurial) glia form a sheath around the surface of the brain (Fig. 7A). Cortex glia are located in the brain cortex and form a tightly-nit three-dimensional scaffold that encapsulates neuronal cell bodies, ganglion mother cells and neuroblasts (Fig. 7B). Neuropile glia surround the neuropile and form septa around individual neuropile compartments, as well as major tracts of neurites (Fig. 7C). Surface glial cells, interconnected by septate junctions and covered by a thick basement membrane, act as the blood-brain barrier (Fig. 7D).[43] Cortex glia fulfill important trophic roles for neuronal cell bodies.[44] In the larval brain,

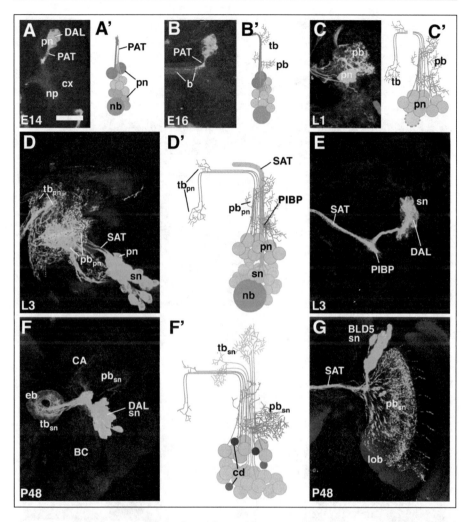

Figure 6. Morphogenesis and branching of neural lineages. A-G are Z-projections of confocal stacks of brains in which individual lineages were labeled by the FLP/FRT induced activation of tau-lacZ (green). For each panel (except G), a representative of the dorso-anterior-lateral (DAL) group of lineages was selected. G shows the baso-lateral-dorsal (BLD) lineage #5. The neuropile is labeled with anti-DN-cadherin (red). In A-D, lineages were labeled by activating FLP in early embryo (primary lineages, A-C; primary plus secondary lineage, D). In E-G, activation of FLP occurred after hatching, resulting in labeling of secondary component of lineage only. A'-F' schematically depict one lineage at the stage corresponding to the adjacent confocal images. Primary neurons are in lilac, secondary neurons in orange. A, A': Stage 14 embryo; B, B': Stage 16 embryo; C, C': early larva; D,D' and E: late larva; F, F' and G: pupa/adult. Abbreviations: b neurite branches; BC baso-central compartment; CA centro-anterior compartment; cd cell death; cx cortex; eb ellipsoid body; lob lobula neuropile; nb neuroblast; np neuropile; PAT primary axon tract; pb proximal branches; PIBP proximal interstitial branchpoint; pn primary neuron; SAT secondary axon tract; sn secondary neuron; tb terminal branches. Bar: 20μm

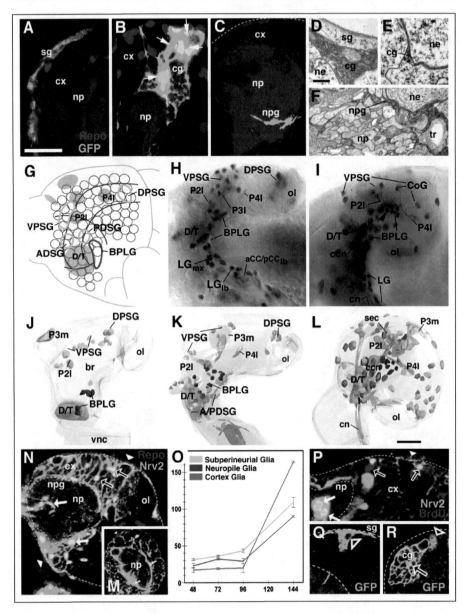

Figure 7. Origin and proliferation of glial cells of the *Drosophila* brain. A-C) Structure of larval glia. GFP labeled clones (induced shortly after hatching) in late larval brain. All three panels show Z-projections of frontal confocal sections of late larval brain hemisphere in which glial clone appears in green. In A and B, glial nuclei are labeled by antiRepo (red); in C, neuropile is labeled by antiSyntaxin (red). A) Surface glia (sg). B) cortex glia (cg). C) neuropile glia (npg). D-F) TEM sections of early larval brains. D) glial sheath at the brain surface. Underneath the relatively electron-translucent surface glia (sg) appears a second layer formed by the surface lamella of the electron-dense cortex glia (cg). Cortex glia, rather than surface glia, contacts neurons (ne) and neuroblasts of the cortex at most locations. E) Brain cortex; cortex glial lamella (cg) appears as electron dense layer in between neurons (ne). Legend coninued on following page.

Figure 7, continued from previous page. F) Cortex-neuropile boundary, showing prominent, electron-dense neuropile glial sheath (npg) separating neuronal somata (ne) from bundles of neurites that constitute the neuropile (np). Tracheae and tracheoles (tr) penetrating the neuropile are always associated with glial sheaths. (G-L) Embryonic origin of brain glia. G) Schematic map of stage 11 embryonic head showing approximate location of the clusters of glia progenitors (outlined in green and red, respectively) in relation to Fas-positive neuropile pioneer clusters (orange) and the brain neuroblast map.[2] Glia progenitors giving rise to surface and cortex glia comprise a dorsal protocerebral cluster (DPSG), ventral protocerebral cluster (VPSG), anterior deuterocerebral cluster (ADSG) and posterior deuterocerebral cluster (PDSG). Neuropile glia (longitudinal glia) is derived from a single cluster (BPLG) located in the deuterocerebral neuromere. H, I) lateral view of heads of embryos labeled with antiRepo expressed in glia cell nuclei (brown) and antiFas II expressed in pioneer neurons and their axons (P2l, P3l, P4l, D/T, aCC/pCC; purple). H) late stage 12. Precursors of neuropile glia, forming the BPLG cluster, migrate dorsally along the cervical connectives, pioneered by the D/T and P2 clusters. Ventrally, cells of the BPLG have linked up with longitudinal glia cells of the ventral nerve cord (LGmx, LGlb: longitudinal glia derived from the maxillary and labial neuromere, respectively). Two major clusters located in the ventral (*VPSG*) and dorsal (*DPSG*) part of the protocerebrum include precursors of surface glia and cortex glia. I) Late stage 14. Neuropile glia (LG and BPLG) form a continuous covering of cervical connective (*ccn*) and connective of ventral nerve cord (*cn*). Note group of small sized cells at dorsal front of BPLG (arrowhead); these cells most likely represent early postmitotic glia cells produced by the proliferating BPLG cluster. Surface glia precursors derived from the VPSG cluster have spread over the lateral and dorsal brain hemisphere. At this stage cortex glia cells (CoG), also derived from the VPSG and DPSG clusters, are seen separately from the more superficial surface glia. J-L) Digital 3D models of brain hemispheres of stage 11 (J), late stage 12 (K) and late stage 14 (L) embryos, illustrating the pattern of different populations of glia cell precursors in lateral view (see color key at top of panel O) note that cortex glial cells (dark green) as entities different from subperineurial glia (light green) are indicated only in the late stage 14 brain (L) because they cannot be distinguished earlier. Structures of the neuropile, including cervical connective (*ccn*), subesophageal commissure (*sco*), supraesophageal commissure (*sec*) and FasII positive clusters [P1, P2l, P3m, P3l, P4l, optic lobe (ol); all shaded grey] are indicated as points of reference. (M-R) Glial proliferation during larval stages. M and N show confocal sections of larval brain hemispheres (M:48h AEL, first instar; N) 144h AEL, late third instar) in which glial nuclei are labeled with antiRepo (red) and glial processes are marked with Nrv2-GFP (green). Arrowheads point at representative surface glial nuclei; open arrows at cortex glia, solid arrows at neuropile glia. Note dramatic increase in all three subclasses of glia between first and third instar. O) Plot of glial cell number against time (in hours after egg laying). P) Confocal section of brain of late larva that had been fed BrdU containing medium for 12h prior to dissection. BrdU incorporation appears in secondary neural lineages, as well as in all three classes of glial cells (arrowheads: surface glia; open arrows: cortex glia; solid arrows: neuropile glia). (Q, R) GFP labeled clones of secondary lineages (neuroblasts indicated by open arrowheads) with adjacent glial cells in third larval instar brains. Q shows surface glia (sg) forming part of secondary lineage (arrowhead). In R, cortex glia (cg; open arrow) is located directly adjacent to secondary lineage (arrowhead). Other abbreviations: cx cortex; np neuropile; ol optic lobe Bars: 20μm (A-C); 0.5μm (D-F); 10μm (G-L)

the meshwork of cortex glial processes ("trophospongium") is required for stabilizing the position of neurons in the cortex and for extension of secondary axon tracts.[7] Neuropile and surface glia play numerous roles in axon pathfinding and targeting.[45-48] Glial septa formed by neuropile glia are essential to establish and stabilize neuropile compartments, such as the glomeruli formed by neurites of olfactory receptors and interneurons in the antennal lobe.[49]

The glial cells of the early larval brain (primary glia) arise from a small number of neuro-glioblasts that are active during the embryonic period. Neuro-glioblasts of the ventral nerve cord have been identified on a single cell basis,[32,33] a feat not yet achieved for the brain. Here, precursors of neuropile glia form a prominent cluster, the baso-posterior cluster, (BPLG)[50] that consists of approximately 20 cells and is located at the base of the brain primordium (Fig. 7G,J). During late embryogenesis, these cells spread out dorsally along the inner surface of the extending neuropile. Precursors of

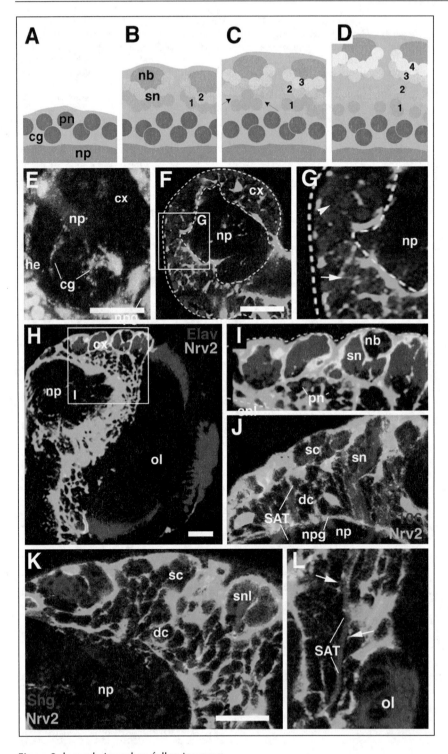

Figure 8, legend viewed on following page.

Figure 8, viewed on previous page. Formation of the trophospongium by cortex glia. A-D) Schematic cross section of brain cortex at different larval stages (A: 1st instar; B 2nd instar; C early 3rd instar; D late 3rd instar), illustrating formation of the trophospongium. Cortex glial cells (cg) are in green, neuroblasts (nb) and secondary neurons (sn) in shades of orange, primary neurons (pn) in lilac, neuropile (np) in gray. Numbers 1-4 indicate birth order of secondary neurons (1: early; 4: late). E) Z-projection of serial horizontal confocal sections of embryonic brain hemisphere in which glial cells are labeled green by GFP reporter construct activated by the *gcm*-Gal4 driver. Neuropile (np) is labeled with antiDN cadherin antibody (red. Cortex glia (cg) is represented by slender, radial cells extending throughout the cortex (cx) from the neuropile (np) to the brain surface. Hemocytes (he) surrounding brain also express *gcm*-gal. 4 (F-I) Confocal sections of brain hemispheres of first instar (F,G) and late third instar (H,I). Glial cells are labeled (green) by GFP reporter activated by the *nrv2*-Gal4 driver. Neurons are labeled by anti-Elav antibody (red). By the first instar, cortex glia have formed a meshwork of lamelliform processes that form more (arrow) or less (arrowhead) complete sheaths around primary neurons. At later stages (H, I) all primary neurons (pn) and the first born secondary neurons (located deep in the cortex) are individually surrounded by glial sheaths; secondary neuroblasts (nb) and their latest progeny (sn) located near the brain surface are enclosed within large glial chambers. J) Confocal section of cortex of late third instar brain labeled with antiBP106 (red, marks secondary lineages) and *nrv2*-Gal4 driving GFP (green; glia). Secondary lineages (sn) and their axon tracts (SAT) are encapsulated by cortex glia. (K,L) Confocal section of cortex of late third instar larval brain labeled with antiShg (DE-cadherin; red) and nrv2-Gal4 driving GFP. DE-cadherin is expressed in secondary neuroblasts and the latest born neurons (snl in K), as well as the SAT formed by these cells. Note enclosure of the Shg-positive cells in large, undivided glial chambers ("superficial chambers"; sc); earlier born neurons located in deep cortex are individually surrounded by glial septa ("deep chambers"; dc). Cortex glial septa (arrows in L) also flank the SAT in deep cortex. Other abbreviations: npg, neuropile glia; ol, optic lobe. Bars: 20 μm

surface glia (approximately 25-30 in the hatching larva) and cortex glia (approximately 10) also originate in a small number of discrete clusters which migrate outward to populate the entire brain (Fig. 7H,I,K,L).[50] This pattern suggests that, similar to what has been found in the ventral nerve cord, glial cells are produced by only few neuro-glioblasts.

Glial cell numbers increase slowly during the first half of larval development, but show a rapid incline in the third larval instar. Overall, glial cell numbers increases from about 30 to more than 100 for surface glia, from 10 to 160 for cortex glia and from 20 to about 90 for neuropile glia (Fig. 7M-O).[51] This increase in cell number is at least in part due to the mitotic divisions of glial cells. Thus, feeding BrdU to larvae at different stages results in clusters of labeled cells that include all three types of glial cells (Fig. 7P). Moreover, a small fraction of late larval glial cells can always be seen in mitosis using a marker that labels phosphorylated histone H3. However, the low frequency of phospho-histone positive glial cells, as well as the finding that glial cells labeled by clonal induction were almost always in close contact with neural lineages (Fig. 7Q,R), indicates that the bulk of added glial cells stems from the proliferation of secondary neuro-glioblasts located at the brain surface. This is also supported by the shape of the glial growth curve, which is almost horizontal during early larval life (when neuroblasts are mitotically quiescent) and becomes steep during the third instar when neuroblasts divide (Fig. 7O).

The trophospongium is formed by cortex glial cells, highly branched and lamellated cells whose processes undergo extensive rearrangements during development (schematically shown in Fig. 8A-D). Cortex glia appear in the stage 16 embryo as elongated, radially oriented cells most of which extend from the brain surface to the neuropile (Fig. 8E).[51,52] Subsequently lateral processes are formed, leading up to the three-dimensional, honey-combed structure revealed by the larval clones shown in Figure 7B. Shortly after hatching these processes are still modest, forming relatively large chambers that enclose multiple primary neurons (Fig. 8F,G). At subsequent stages, process density increases, so that by the second instar each primary neuron is completely enclosed by cortex glia. Cortex glia also form a superficial lamella that extends underneath the surface glial layer. Thus, from the second instar onward, the glial layer covering the brain is composed of an outer, electron-light lamella of surface glia and an inner, extremely thin and electron-dense lamella formed by cortex glia (Fig. 7D).

Beginning with the second instar, dividing neuroblasts produce secondary neurons that form an outer cortex of increasing thickness around the inner layer of primary neurons. During this phase, the growth of the trophospongium and neuroblast proliferation must be coordinated in a complex manner. Close to the brain surface, individual chambers of the trophospongium are large, containing a neuroblast, undivided ganglion mother cells and 20 to 40 neurons (Fig. 8C,D,H-K). Each superficial trophospongium chamber corresponds to part of one secondary lineage, such that the neurons newly formed by one neuroblast over a certain period of time are "received" into one chamber, thereby isolating them from other lineages. At deeper levels, chambers become smaller, such that older secondary neurons (like primary neurons before) become individually enclosed by glia. This implies that there is a dynamic rearrangement of glia processes at the transition zone from large chambers to small chambers.

Tracheal System of the Brain

Gas exchange in the insect body is mediated by a branched network of air-filled tubes called tracheae. In the brain and ventral nerve cord, tracheae form an anastomosing plexus at the cortex-neuropile surface (perineuropilar plexus).[53] From this plexus, several branches sprout into the neuropile and the cortex (see below). Tracheae develop from a bilateral set of metameric invaginations of the embryonic ectoderm.[54] Each tracheal invagination subsequently forms a stereotyped set of primary branches (Fig. 9A). One branch, called ganglionic branch (GB), grows towards each neuromere of the ventral nerve cord in the late embryo (Fig. 9B, arrowhead "1").[55] Advancing medially, GBs pass underneath the neuropile of the ventral nerve cord (Fig. 9B, arrowhead "2") and then form a 180-degree turn around the medial and dorsal surface of the neuropile (arrowhead "3" and "4"). During larval stages, the advancing tips of the GBs close the circle and fuse with a more proximal part of the same or adjacent GBs. A similar pattern of ring- (or noose-) shaped tracheae is generated in the brain. Here, one main trachea, the cerebral trachea (CT), branches off the first tracheal invagination in segment T2 (Fig. 9A). After reaching the medial surface of the brain neuropile in the embryo (Fig. 9B, arrowhead "5") the CT gives off multiple branches (the primary tracheae of the brain) that grow laterally and medially around the neuropile surface to eventually meet and fuse.

Figure 9C-G show Z-projections of confocal sections that illustrate the growth of the tracheal network in the larval brain. Panels 8H-K show the tracheal system of an early third instar brain (when all primary and secondary branches are in place) in the form of 3D digital models. In the late embryo the cerebral trachea is visible as a thick, posteriorly directed branch of the first segmental trachea that belongs to the second thoracic segment (Fig. 9C,D). The CT follows the medial surface of the brain where the neuropile is covered by a layer of surface glia (Fig. 9C). The cerebral trachea and all of its branches are embedded in a glial layer. During the first larval instar, all of the primary brain tracheae become established. First, around the time of hatching, the CT splits into a laterally and a ventrally directed trunk (Fig. 9D,E). By the beginning of the second instar (48h after egg laying, AEL; Fig. 9F), the lateral trunk gives rise to the centro-medial trachea (CMT), centro-posterior trachea (CPT) and baso-lateral trachea (BLT). The ventral trunk bifurcates into the baso-medial trachea (BMT) and the lateral and medial baso-central trachea (BCTl, BCTm).

By the early third instar two to three secondary tracheae enter the center of the neuropile. They include the trachea of the mushroom body (TMB), the trachea of the antennocerebral tract (TAC) and the internal dorsal transverse trachea (DT; not always found). The mushroom body trachea in most cases branches off the BCT trachea. The trachea of the antennocerebral tract (TAC) typically constitutes a branch of the CPTm trachea. In addition to the TAC and TMB tracheae which are directed inward, into the center of the neuropile, a number of secondary tracheal branches project outward into the cortex and the optic lobe (Fig. 9).

Although the main, primary tracheal branches described above can be recognized faithfully in all brains, the higher order branching pattern is highly variable. For example, the secondary trachea towards the mushroom body (TMB) may branch off the BCTm in one hemisphere and the CPT in the other hemisphere of the same brain. This is similar to the reported variability in higher order branching patterns of epidermal tracheae and strikingly contrasts with the invariant pattern of neuroblasts, neurons and axon tracts in the brain.

Neuroanatomy of the Developing *Drosophila* Brain: The Systems of Lineages, Tracts and Compartments

Pattern of Primary Pioneer Tracts

As described in section 'Secondary Neuroblasts and GMCs of the Larval Brain' of this chapter, the brain of the late embryo is formed by approximately 100 lineages per side whose neurons adhere to each other and, at the onset of neuropile formation (stage 13), appear as cone shaped clusters distributed rather evenly over the periphery of the brain (Fig. 10A). Axons formed by neurons of the same lineage typically form one bundle, the primary axon tract (PAT; Fig. 10A, B, C). The pattern of PATs appears highly invariant and provides essential information about the structure of the evolving neuropile (see section 'Synopsis of Lineages, Compartments and Fiber Tracts of the Larval Brain' below). To describe the pattern of primary lineages and their PATs, a scaffold of pioneer axon tracts laid down by early born neurons of a subset of lineages has been utilized.[52,56,57] We will first introduce the pattern of pioneer tracts, to then relate the primary and secondary lineages to this pattern. Fig. 10D shows the FasII-positive pioneer neurons in relationship to neuromere boundaries, visualized by an engrailed-lacZ reporter construct; panel 10E is a schematic map of pioneer neurons in the late embryonic brain.

Longitudinal pioneer tracts: Three longitudinal tracts (connectives) pioneer the neuropile of the ventral nerve cord.[56,58] By the end of embryogenesis, each of these three connectives has split into a dorsal and ventral component.[56-58] The connectives of the ventral nerve cord continue anteriorly into the two preoral neuromeres that form the basal brain, the tritocerebrum and deuterocerebrum (Fig. 10E).[56,59,60] The medial connective continues as the medial cervical tract (MCT); the intermediate connective as the lateral cervical tracts (LCT) and the lateral connective as the posterior cervical tract (PCT), respectively. The MCT is organized by the large D/T pioneer cluster, located in the deutero-tritocerebral boundary region. Ascending D/T axons reach the P2 clusters, located in the antero-dorsal deuterocerebrum, that pioneer the ventral fascicle of the supraesophageal commissure (vSEC; Fig. 10E). The LCT is formed by axons of D/T and P1 that extend laterally adjacent of the MCT. Three tracts to and from the "corner points" of the basal brain converge upon P1. The horizontally directed baso-medial protocerebral tract (BMPT) connects posterior and anterior realms of the basal brain (P1 to/from P4m). The centro-anterior protocerebral tract (CAPT) and dorso-posterior protocerebral tract (DPPT) originate from the P3c and P3m clusters, respectively, both located in the boundary region between deuterocerebrum and protocerebrum (shaded light blue in Fig. 10E).

Transverse pioneer tract: The dorsal and lateral protocerebrum consists of lineages whose PATs form transverse (commissural) fiber systems connecting the two brain hemispheres. These transverse systems are quite separate from the longitudinally oriented MCT, LCT and PCT systems and are pioneered by the lateral protocerebral tract (LPT). The LPT is formed by several medio-laterally arranged clusters of pioneer neurons (P5l, P4l, P3l) that extend from the optic lobe primordium (OL) to the dorsal midline, where they establish the dorsal fascicle of the supraesophageal commissure (dSEC in Fig. 10E).

Mushroom body: The massive fiber tract formed by the mushroom body neurons (MB) interconnects the posterior protocerebrum with the proto-deuterocerebral boundary domain. This tract (peduncle; indicated by gray hatched line in Fig. 10E) converges upon the P1 cluster, but then makes a sharp turn medially, pioneering the medial lobe of the mushroom body.

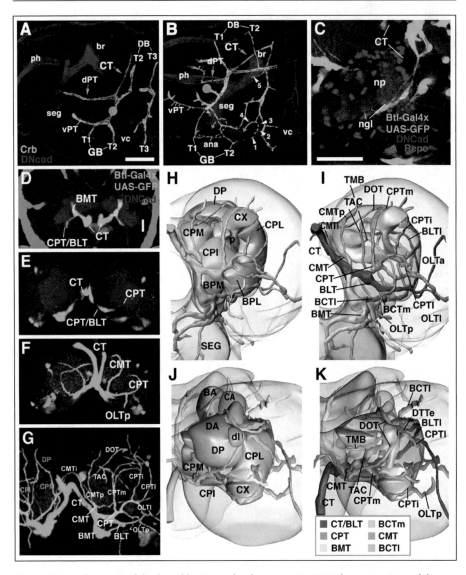

Figure 9. Development of the larval brain tracheal system. (A, B) Embryonic origin of the cerebral trachea and ganglionic tracheal branches. Both panels show Z-projections of confocal sections of embryos (lateral view, anterior to the left) labeled with antiCrb (green) to visualize tracheae. AntiDN-cadherin (red) labels neuropile and other embryonic structures. A) Stage 14. Cerebral trachea (CT) and dorsal pharyngeal trachea (dPT) form a Y-shaped, anteriorly directed branch of the first segmental trachea (I) that grow around the posterior surface of the brain (br). Other branches of the first segmental trachea are the dorsal branches (DB) of segments T2 and T1 (formed later than stage 14), the ventral ganglionic branches (GB) of segments T1 and T2 and the ventral pharyngeal trachea. The location of the anterior spiracle is indicated by violet circle. B) Stage 15 late. Segmental tracheae have fused, primary branches have increased in length and some secondary branches have been initiated. Note position of the cerebral trachea (CT) and dorsal pharyngeal trachea (dPT). The cerebral trachea has reached the medial surface of the brain neuropile (arrowhead "5"). Legend continued on following page.

Figure 9, continued from previous page. Ventral ganglionic branches contact the ventral surface of the neuropile of the ventral nerve cord (vc; arrowhead "1"). During later stages ganglionic branches will extend underneath the neuropile, turn dorsally (hatched blue line; arrowheads "2" and "3") and then laterally (solid blue line, arrowhead "4"). Anastomoses (ana; gray hatched line) will interconnect ganglionic branches of neighboring segments. C) Z-projection of a confocal stack of brain of late embryo in which tracheae are visualized by the expression of *btl*-Gal4 driving UAS-GFP (green); the neuropile is labeled with antiDN-cadherin (red) and glial cells are labeled by antiRepo (blue). (D-G) Z-projections of confocal stacks of brains of stage 16 embryo (D), first instar larva (E), second instar larva (F) and early third instar larva (G). Tracheae are visualized by the expression of *btl*-Gal4 driving UAS-GFP (green); the neuropile is labeled with antiDN-cadherin (red). (H-K) Digital 3D models of right brain hemisphere showing neuropile compartments in grey and major tracheae in different colors. Models of the top row (H,I) represent posterior view (dorsal up, lateral to the right); second row (I,K) shows dorsal view (dorsal up, lateral to the right). In models of left column (H, J), coloring indicates depth of tracheae: Tracheae forming the perineuropilar plexus (surrounding the neuropile surface) are depicted in green; secondary branches turning externally into the cortex of the central brain are shown in light blue; optic lobe tracheae in purple. Two secondary branches turning centrally into the neuropile are shown in red. In models of right column (H,K) neuropile is also semi-transparent and each primary brain trachea together with its belonging secondary branches is depicted in its own color (see color key at bottom of panel), which allows one to follow the trajectories of tracheae. For description of pattern of tracheae see text. Abbreviations: BA baso-anterior (antennal) neuropile compartment; BC baso-central neuropile compartment; BAT baso-anterior trachea; BCT baso-central trachea; BCTl lateral baso-central trachea; BCTm medial baso-central trachea; BCvT baso-cervical trachea; BLT baso-lateral trachea; BLTl lateral branch of baso-lateral trachea; BPL baso-posterior lateral neuropile compartment; BMT baso-medial trachea; BPM baso-posterior medial neuropile compartment; CA centro-anterior neuropile compartment; CMT centro-medial trachea; CMTa anterior branch of centro-medial trachea; CMTi intermediate branch of centro-medial trachea; CMTp posterior branch of centro-medial trachea; CPI centro-posterior intermediate neuropile compartment; CPL centro-posterior lateral neuropile compartment; CPM centro-posterior medial compartment; CPT centro-posterior trachea; CPTm medial branch of centroposterior trachea; CPTi intermediate branch of centro-posterior trachea; CPTl lateral branch of centro-posterior trachea; CT cerebral trachea; CX calyx of mushroom body; DA dorso-anterior neuropile compartment; dl dorsal lobe of mushroom body; DP dorso-posterior compartment; DOT dorsal oblique trachea; ml medial lobe of mushroom body; DTTe external dorsal transverse trachea; DTTi internal dorsal transverse trachea; INT intraneuropilat tracheae of ventral nerve cord; ngl neuropile glia; OLTa anterior optic lobe trachea; OLTl lateral optic lobe trachea; OLTp posterior optic lobe trachea; p peduncle of mushroom body; ph pharynx; PNP$_{br}$ perineuropilar plexus of brain; PNP$_{vc}$ perineuropilear plexus of ventral nerve cord; SEG subesophageal neuropile; SET subesophageal tracheae; sp spur of mushroom body; TAC trachea of the antenno-cerebral tract; ThT thoracic trachea; TMB trachea of the mushroom body. Bars: 20 μm

Pattern of Lineages and Their Axon Tracts

Primary lineages and PATs: Marking the evolving neuropile of late embryos with global markers such as Synaptobrevin-GFP fusion protein driven by *elav*-Gal4 reveals that PATs are rather uniformly directed away from the surface and extend centripetally towards the center of the brain primordium (Figs. 10A,B; 11A).[17,38,52] As a result, the direction of most PATs correlates with the location of the corresponding primary lineage. PATs of lineages located at the posterior pole of the brain primordium project anteriorly, those of dorsal lineages ventrally and so on. PATs line up with the neuropile pioneer tracts in whose vicinity they are located. Thus, for example, lineages grouped around P3c align their PATs with the CAPT tract; posterior lineages close to P4m project PATs close to the pioneer tract (BMPT) formed by this cluster and so on. Figs. 11 and 12 show the pattern of primary lineages and PATs.

Compartments: Up to stage 15, PATs consist of mostly short, unbranched axons that converge in the center of the brain primordium (Fig. 10A). The assembly of PATs represents the "nucleus"

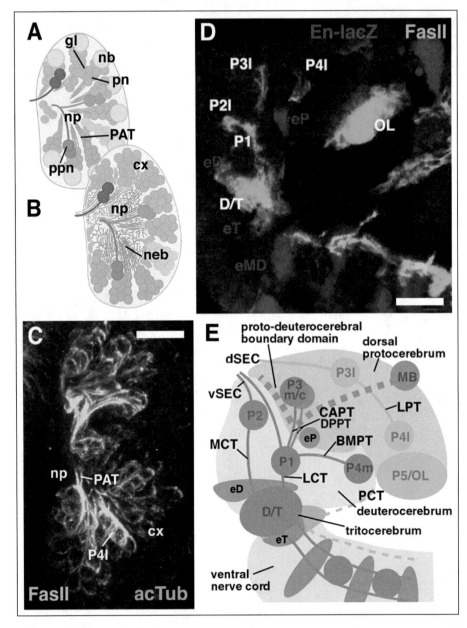

Figure 10. Patterning of the brain neuropile. A,B) Schematic horizontal sections of brain hemisphere illustrating neuropile formation. Neuroblasts (nb) produce lineages comprising precursors of primary neurons (pn) and glial cells (gl). At the stage shown in A (stage 13-15 of embryonic development) primary neurons have formed short axon stumps organized in bundles, with each bundle belonging to one lineage (primary axon bundle, PAT). Early differentiating neurons (neuropile pioneers; ppn) establish scaffold of pioneer tracts. Primary axon tracts orient themselves around the pioneer tracts and form the early nucleus of the neuropile (np). Legend continued on following page.

Figure 10, continued from previous page. Branching of primary axons (neb; stage 16-17; B) leads to an increase in neuropile volume. C) Confocal horizontal section of stage 13 embryonic brain hemisphere double labeled with anti-Acetylated tubulin (all differentiating neurons; yellow) and antiFasII (neuropile pioneers, green). Primary axon bundles (PAT) converge radially towards the center of the brain. Note, at this confocal level, anteriorly directed axon bundles, emanating from lineages localized in the posterior cortex and extending parallel to the fasII-positive P4l pioneer neurons. D) Z-projection of confocal parasagittal sections of stage 13 embryonic brain double-labeled with antiFasII (pioneer tracts; green) and an engrailed *(rhx25)*-lacZ reporter construct (red). Engrailed expression domains demarcate the posterior boundary of the deuterocerebrum (eD), the tritocerebrum (eT) and the mandibular segment (eMD). The small engrailed-positive "head spot" (eP) indicates a point located on the otherwise undefined protocerebral-deuterocerebral boundary. E) Schematic lateral view of embryonic brain (anterior to the left; dorsal to the top), showing FasII positive pioneer tracts in relationship to dorso-ventral and antero-posterior axis and to neuromere boundaries. Other abbreviations: BMPT baso-medial protocerebral tract; CAPT central anterior protocerebral tract; cx cortex; DPPT dorso-posterior protocerebral tract; dSEC dorsal supraesophageal commissure; dSEC dorsal supraesophageal commissure; D/T deutero/tritocerebral FasII cluster; LCT lateral cervical tract; LPT lateral protocerebral tract; MB mushroom body; MCT medial cervical tract; OL optic lobe; P1, P2, P3l/m/c, P4m/l, P5 FasII positive pioneer clusters; PCT posterior cervical tract; vSEC ventral supraesophageal commissure. Bars: 20 μm

from which the brain neuropile is formed. Neuropile formation proceeds by branching of the PATs (Fig. 10B; see also Fig. 6B). These axonal and dendritic branches make up the content of the emerging neuropile compartments. Using the reproducible pattern of PATs and FasII-positive neuropile pioneer tracts as landmarks, the discrete neuropile compartments defined for the larval brain can be recognized already in the embryo (Fig. 13A-C; see also section 'Synopsis of Lineages, Compartments and Fiber Tracts of the Larval Brain' below).[52] Between early and late larval instar, compartments grow substantially through additional branching of primary neurons, as well as the "invasion" of the neuropile by SATs (Fig. 13D-I). Branching of secondary lineages, as well as the metamorphic reorganization of primary neurons, lead to changes in compartmental shape and the addition of new (adult-specific) compartments; however, these changes notwithstanding, the basic pattern of neuropile compartments of the larval brain can be followed throughout metamorphosis into the adult brain (Fig. 13J-L).

Secondary lineages and SATs: Primary neurons of the brain and ventral nerve cord form the functional circuitry controlling larval behavior. During the early larval period, the brain grows only slowly, mainly due to increased branching of primary neurons. Starting during the second instar, neuroblasts become reactivated and produce secondary lineages. Similar to primary axons, axons of a given secondary lineage fasciculate with each other, thereby forming a discrete secondary axon tract (SAT) within the brain cortex and neuropile. SATs penetrate the neuropile glial sheath, or travel along the neuropile surface for variable distances (Figs. 11B; 12C).[38] In terms of overall number and trajectory, secondary and primary lineages show many similarities and we have adopted a nomenclature that suggests correspondences between lineages.[38,52] Thus, we assume that, for example, the primary BA lineages are generated by the same neuroblasts that later form the secondary BA lineages. Likewise, PATs of primary BA lineages show similar trajectories than SATs of the larval secondary BA lineages. However, one should point out that lineage tracing and the analysis of molecular markers that are continuously expressed from the embryonic to the late larval period are needed to establish in detail the link between a primary lineage and its secondary counterpart.

Secondary tract systems in the larval and pupal neuropile: Within the neuropile, tracts of several neighboring lineages converge to form larger "secondary tract systems" (Fig. 11C,D).[53] Some secondary tract systems extend along the glial sheaths in between neuropile compartments; others penetrate the center of compartments, typically following the above described pioneer tracts laid down by primary axons at an earlier stage (Fig. 11E).[57] Each secondary lineage forms a tract with an invariant and characteristic trajectory within the neuropile. That is to say, a given SAT reaches

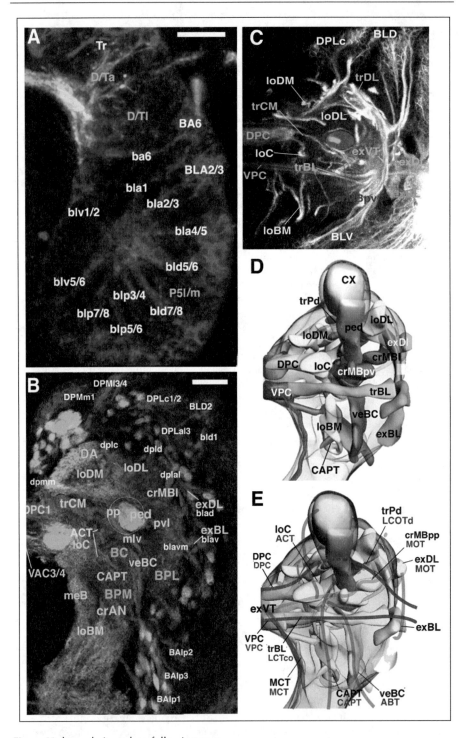

Figure 11, legend viewed on following page.

Figure 11, viewed on previous page. Pattern of lineages and their axon bundles in the embryonic and larval brain. A) Z-projection of horizontal confocal sections of a representative late stage 15 brain hemisphere (lateral to the right), double labeled with antiFasII (green; neuropile pioneer neurons) and UAS-synaptobrevin-GFP driven by *elav*-Gal4 (red; primary lineages). Shown are a subset of lineages of the basal brain. B) Z-projection of frontal confocal sections (lateral to the right) of late larval brain labeled with the BP106 antibody (secondary lineages and their axon tracts; red) and a choline-acetyl transferase-(Chat)-Gal4; UAS-GFP construct (primary neurons and neuropile; green). Subset of lineages and SATs at a central level (level of supraesophageal commissure and medial lobe of mushroom body visible at the left margin of panel) are shown. C) Z-projection prepared from frontal confocal cross sections of BP106 labeled late larval brain. Fiber tracts within the central part of the neuropile (level of supraesophageal commissure), formed by the confluence of secondary axon tracts labeled by antiBP106, were identified on the basis of location and axonal trajectory. D) 3D digital model of larval brain neuropile (posterior view) showing pattern of secondary axon tract systems (posterior view). Surface of neuropile and mushroom body are shaded light and intermediate grey, respectively. Commissural tracts forming the supraesophageal commissure are dark gray. Longitudinal tract systems are colored yellow, transverse systems blue; circumferential systems around mushroom body (lobes, peduncle) are red; circumferential systems around antennal lobe (BA compartment) are olive; external systems (at neuropile surface) are bright green; medial cervical tract is violet. E) Spatial relationship of secondary axon tract systems to primary systems, laid down in the embryo. 3D digital model of brain neuropile (grey) in posterior view. Secondary tract systems are rendered in light blue. Red lines schematically indicate the trajectory of primary axon tracts in the late larval brain as visualized by antiFasII.[57] Secondary tract systems are annotated in black letters, primary systems in red. Note that the majority of secondary tract systems follows the flow of primary axon tracts. Abbreviations: ABT, antero-basal tracts (= crAN, veBC et al); ACT antenno-cerebral tract; BA, baso-anterior lineages; BAlp, baso-anterior lineages, postero-lateral subgroup; BC, basal central compartment; BLA, basal lateral anterior lineages; BLAd, anterior baso-lateral lineages, dorsal subgroup; BLAv, ventral baso-lateral lineages, ventral subgroup; BLAvm, anterior baso-lateral lineages, ventromedial subgroup; BLD, dorsal baso-lateral lineages; BLP, basal lateral posterior lineages; BLV, basal lateral ventral lineages; BLVa, ventral baso-lateral lineages, anterior subgroup; BPL, basal postero-lateral compartment; BPM, basal postero-medial compartment; CAPT, centro-anterior protocerebral tract; crAN, circumferential tracts of antennal lobe; crMB, circumferential tracts of the mushroom body (l lateral; mlv, ventral of medial lobe; pp, around proximal peduncle; pv, ventral of peduncle; pvl, ventro-lateral of peduncle); CX, calyx of mushroom body; DA, dorsal anterior compartment; DPC, dorso-posterior commissures; DPLal, lateral dorso-posterior lineages, antero-lateral subgroup; DPLc, lateral dorso-posterior lineages, central subgroup; DPLd, lateral dorso-posterior lineages, dorsal subgroup; DPMl, medial dorso-posterior lineages, lateral subgroup; DPMm, medial dorso-posterior lineages, medial subgroup; DPMpm, medial dorso-posterior lineages, postero-medial subgroup; D/Ta, D/Tl, complex of pioneer clusters at deutero/tritocerebral boundary; exBL, external baso-lateral tract system; exDL, external dorso-lateral tract system; exVT, external vertical tract system; LCOTd, lateral commissural optic tract (= trPd); LCTco, commissural component of LCT (= trBL); loBM, baso-medial longitudinal tract system; loC, central longitudinal tract system (= ACTet al); loDL, longitudinal dorso-lateral tract system; loDM, dorso-medial longitudinal tract system; meB, median bundle; MCT, medial cervical tract (= meB); MOT, medial optic tract (= exBL, crMBpp et al); ped, peduncle of mushroom body; P5l/m, ventral protocerebral pioneer neuron cluster; Tr, tritocerebral lineages; trBL, transverse baso-lateral tract system; trCM, transverse centro-medial tract system; trDL, transverse dorso-lateral tract system; trPd, transverse postero-dorsal tract system; VAC, ventro-anterior commissures; veBC, vertical baso-central tract system; VPC, ventro-posterior commissures. Bars: 20 μm

the neuropile at a characteristic position and then joins one or more (in case the tract branches) secondary tract systems.

Secondary neurons differentiate during the pupal period, sending out proximal and terminal branches that form synapses. Most of the secondary tract systems formed by secondary lineages in the larva remain visible throughout the pupal period and evolve into the long fiber tracts that have

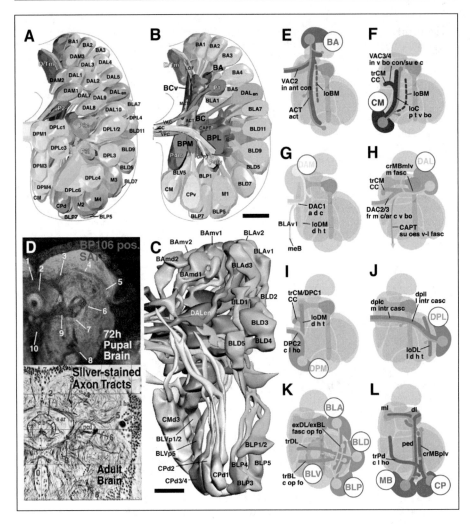

Figure 12. Neural lineages of the brain and their projection patterns. (A,B) 3D digital models of one late embryonic brain hemisphere. Landmark structures shown in gray are the outline of the brain and the FasII-positive neuropile pioneer clusters (D/T, P1, P2l, P3m/l, P4m/l). Different groups of primary lineages and compartments are rendered in different colors. A shows a dorsal view of right hemisphere; medial to the left, anterior to the top. In B, cell bodies of lineages of dorsal hemisphere (DAM, DAL, DPM, DPL) are omitted to show ventral lineages (BA, CM, BLA, BLD, BLP, BLV), as well as emerging neuropile in the center of the brain. C) Model of secondary lineages of late larval brain. Similar to the embryonic brain hemisphere shown in panel B, dorsal lineages are omitted and only basal lineages are shown, following the same color code as in B. D) Correspondence between pupal secondary axon tracts and adult fiber tracts (frontal views; ventral to the bottom). Photograph at the top shows Z-projection of confocal sections of pupal brain (72h apf) labeled with antiBP106 (red, labels secondary axon tracts) and antiDN-cadherin (green, labels neuropile compartments). Photograph at the bottom shows section of adult brain (from http://web. neurobio.arizona.edu/Flybrain/html/atlas/silver/frontal/index.html) where fibers are visualized through silver impregnation. Numbers 1-10 point out specific BP106-positive pupal tracts and adult fiber bundles with highly similar topology. Legend continued on following page.

Figure 12, continued from previous page. E-L) Topography of major fiber systems formed by the different groups of lineages. Each panel schematically shows dorsal view of one brain hemisphere in which mushroom body (mb) and compartments are shaded gray. In each panel, location of group of primary lineages is depicted as a lightly colored circle; the corresponding secondary lineage group is shown as darkly colored domain surrounding sphere. Similarly, trajectories of PATs formed by primary neurons are shown in light color, SATs are rendered in dark colors. Note close spatial relationship between primary and secondary lineage tracts. Most fiber systems are annotated with two different abbreviations. The upper one corresponds to the name introduced for the larval tracts.[38] The lower abbreviation refers to the name of a tract in the adult fly brain[26] that we propose develops from the corresponding larval fiber system shown here. Abbreviations: act, antenno-cerebral tract; a d c, antero-dorsal commissure; ar c v bo, commissure of ventral body; BA, basal anterior lineages and baso-anterior compartment; BAmd, basal anterior lineages, medio-dorsal subgroup; BAmv, basal anterior lineages, medio-ventral subgroup; BC, baso-central compartment; BCv, baso-cervical compartment; BLA, basal lateral anterior lineages; BLAd, basal lateral anterior lineages, dorsal subgroup; BLAv, basal lateral anterior lineages, ventral subgroup; BLD, basal lateral dorsal lineages; BLP, basal lateral posterior lineages; BLV, basal lateral ventral lineages; BLVp, basal lateral ventral lineages, posterior subgroup; BPL, baso-posterior lateral compartment; BPM, baso-posterior medial compartment; CAPT, centro-anterior protocerebral tract; cc, primordium of central complex; c l ho, commissure of lateral horn; CM, central medial lineages; CMd, central medial lineages, dorsal subgroup; c op fo, commissure of the optic foci; CPd, central posterior dorsal lineages; CPd, central posterior ventral lineages, dorsal subgroup; CPv, central posterior ventral lineages, ventral subgroup; crMBmlv, circumferential tracts of the mushroom body, ventral of medial lobe; DAC, dorso-anterior commissures; DAL, dorsal anterior lateral lineages; DAM, dorsal anterior medial lineages; DC, dorsal commissure; d h t, dorsal horizontal tract; dl, dorsal lobe of mushroom body; DPC, dorso-posterior commissures; DPL, dorsal posterior lateral lineages; DPLc, dorsal central lateral lineages; dlplc/dpll central fascicles of dorso-posterior lateral lineages; DPM, dorsal posterior medial lineages; DPPT, dorso-posterior protocerebral tract; D/Tm complex of pioneer clusters at deutero/tritocerebral boundary; eb, ellipsoid body; exBL, external baso-lateral tract system; exDL, external dorso-lateral tract system; fasc op fo, fasciculus of the optic foci; fr m c, frontal medial commissure; in ant con, inter antennal connective; in v bo con, inter ventral body connective; LCT, lateral cervical tract; l d h t, lateral dorsal horizontal tract; l ho, lateral horn; l intr casc, lateral intracerebral cascades; loBM, baso-medial longitudinal tract system; loC, central longitudinal tract system; loDL, longitudinal dorso-lateral tract system; loDM, dorso-medial longitudinal tract system; M, mushroom body lineages; MCT, medial cervical tract; meB, median bundle (= part of MCT); m fasc medial fascicle; m intr, casc medial intracerebral cascades; ml, medial lobe of mushroom body; P1 complex of pioneer clusters in anterior deuterocerebrum; P2 cluster in dorso-medial deuterocerebrum; P3c, pioneer cluster in proto-deuterocerebral boundary domain; P3l, P4lv dorsal protocerebral pioneer clusters; P4m, postero-medial pioneer cluster; P5m ventral, protocerebral pioneer cluster; ped, peduncle of mushroom body; pi, pars intercerebralis; p t v bo, posterior tract of ventral body; s ar, superior arch; su e c, sub-ellipsoid commissure; su oes v-l fasc, subesophageal ventro-lateral protocerebral fascicle; trBL, transverse baso-lateral tract system; trCM, transverse centro-medial tract system; trDL, transverse dorso-lateral tract system; trPd, transverse postero-dorsal tract system; VAC, ventro-anterior commissures; VPC ventro-posterior commissures; Bars: 10 μm (A, B); 20 μm (C)

been identified for the adult brain (Fig. 12D).[26] Therefore, the detailed analysis of secondary axon tracts will eventually allow for a systematic effort to unravel connectivity of the adult brain.

Synopsis of Lineages, Compartments and Fiber Tracts of the Larval Brain

We will provide in the following a brief description of the topology of lineages in the *Drosophila* brain. Lineages were grouped by location and axon tract projection as described in detail in Pereanu and Hartenstein and Younossi-Hartenstein et al.[38,52] A three dimensional model of a fraction of the lineages visible in the late embryo and third-instar larva is depicted in Figure 12A-C. Panels E-L of Figure 12 present schematic sketches depicting the major trajectories of lineages. Some of the tracts that are visible in the larval period can be tentatively assigned to tracts of the adult fly brain

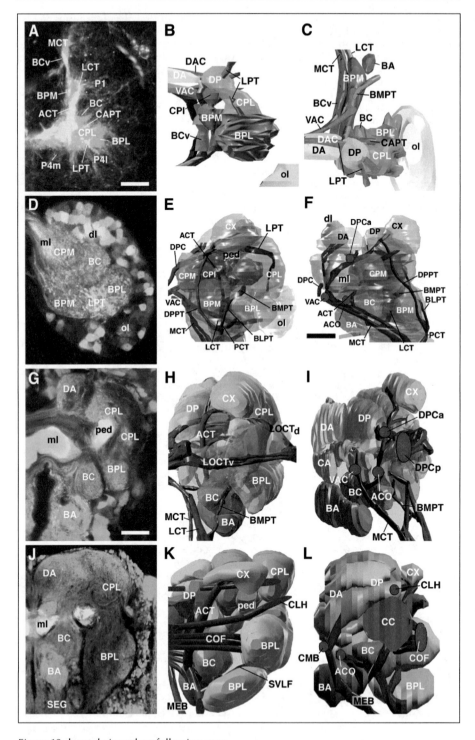

Figure 13, legend viewed on following page.

Figure 13, viewed on previous page. Compartments of the brain neuropile. Each row of panels corresponds to one developmental stage (A-C: Stage 15 embryo; D-F: first instar larva; G-H: late third instar larva; J-L: adult). Panels of left column (A, D, G, J) show Z-projections of confocal sections (A, D: horizontal; G, J: frontal) in which neuropile is labeled green by antiDN-cadherin (A) or ChaT-GFP. The remainder of panels show 3D digital models of compartments in posterior view (middle column; B, E, H, K; lateral to the right) and medial/sagittal view (right column; F, I, L); panel C of right column represents dorsal view (anterior to the top). Each compartment is consistently shown in its own color. FasII-positive tracts are rendered dark grey. In E and F, compartments are rendered semi-transparent to allow for clearer view of tracts. In H, I, K, L, the baso-cervical, baso-posterior medial and centro-posterior medial/centro-posterior intermediate compartments and their adult counterparts are omitted from the models for clarity. In medial views (F, I, L), red ovals demarcate position of commissural tracts. Note formation of central complex compartments (CC in L) that expands within the space flanked by commissures. Abbreviations: ACO, antennal commissure; ACT, antenno-cerebral tract; BA, baso-anterior (antennal) compartment; BC, baso-central compartment; BCv, baso-cervical compartment; BLPT, baso-lateral protocerebral tract; BMPT, baso-medial protocerebral tract; BPL, baso-posterior lateral compartment; BPM, baso-posterior medial compartment; CA, centro-anterior compartment; CAPT, centro-anterior protocerebral tract; CC, central complex; CLH, commissure of the lateral horn; CMB, chiasm of median bundle; COF, great commissures of optic foci; CPI, centro-posterior intermediate compartment; CPL, centro-posterior lateral compartment; CPM, centro-posterior medial compartment; CX, calyx compartment; DA, dorso-anterior compartment; DAC, dorso-anterior commissures; dl, dorsal lobe of mushroom body; DP, dorso-posterior compartment; DPCa, DPCp, anterior and posterior component of dorso-posterior commissures; DPPT, dorso-posterior protocerebral tract; LCT, lateral cervical tract; LOCT$_d$, dorsal larval optic commissural tract; LOCT$_v$, ventral larval optic commissural tract; LPT, lateral protocerebral tract; MCT, medial cervical tract; MEB, median bundle; ml, medial lobe of mushroom body; ol, optic lobe; P1, P4m/l FasII positive pioneer clusters; PCT, posterior cervical tract; ped, peduncle of mushroom body; SEG, subesophageal ganglion; SVLF, sub-esophageal ventro-lateral fascicle; VAC, ventro-anterior commissures; VPC, ventro-posterior commissures. Bars: 10 μm (A-F); 30 μm (G-L)

(Fig. 12D),[26] and in these cases, the term for the larval tract shown in Figure 12E-L is followed by the term describing the corresponding adult tract.

Deuterocerebrum

Primary lineages falling into the realm of the deuterocerebrum, as defined by the expression domain of engrailed, comprise the BA group (Fig. 12A-C,E). It is possible that the CM lineages (Fig. 12A-C,F), located at a postero-medial-basal position, also have a deuterocerebral origin, although this needs to be confirmed by future lineage tracing. The axon bundles formed by these two groups of lineages are oriented preferentially along the antero-posterior axis, BA bundles growing posteriorly, CM bundles anteriorly (Fig. 12E,F). In addition, many BA and CM lineages emit collateral transverse fiber tracts that cross in the brain commissures and/or contribute to the primordium of the central complex (Fig. 12E,F). The BPM compartment appears as an elongated neuropile domain surrounding these deuterocerebral axon tracts (Fig. 13A-F). The BA (= antennal) compartment represents the anterior part of the deuterocerebral neuromere. It evolves as an anterior "alcove" of the BPM, pioneered by the PATs of the medial BA lineages (Figs.12E, 13C,F). Branches of fibers around the MCT tract develop into the BCv compartment (Fig. 13B,C) which is located medial to the BPM.

Major axon tracts formed by BA lineages are the antennocerebral tract that connects the deuterocerebrum to the calyx of the mushroom body and the antennal commissure in between the antennal lobes (BA compartments; Fig. 12E). Both of these connections grow into prominent fiber bundles of the adult brain. The prominent larval loC fiber system, formed by CM lineages as well as BA lineages, most likely gives rise to the posterior tract of the ventral body described for the adult fly brain (Fig. 12E,F).[26] Commissural branches of the loC grow towards the primordium of the central complex (see below) and cross in the commissures closely associated with this structure, called VAC3/4 in the larva and sub-ellipsoid commissure/inter ventral body connective in the adult.[26]

Lineages of the Deutero-Protocerebral Border Region

Two engrailed expressing lineages derived from the engrailed "head spot" define the boundary between deuterocerebrum and protocerebrum in the late embryo and larva (Fig. 12B,C).[52,59] In the late larva, one of these en-positive lineages corresponds to DALv;3 the other one shifts dorsally and forms the DPLam lineage.[38] We define the region flanked by horizontal lines drawn through these two lineages as the "deutero-protocerebral boundary region". Two groups of lineages, DAM and DAL, fall within this boundary region. Axon tracts of the DAM lineages are primarily oriented postero-medially, crossing in the ventral part of the brain commissure; branching of these axons form the major contribution of the CA and DA compartments of the brain (Figs.12G; 13A-C). Among the DAM neurons are some that have axons descending into the subesophageal ganglion via the median bundle (Fig. 12G; see also Fig. 4 for DiI labeled DAM neuron). Larval SATs of the DAM group also form part of the dorsomedian longitudinal tract (loDM) that interconnects anterior and posterior domains within the medial brain (Fig. 12G). This fiber system may well constitute the forerunner of the dorsal horizontal tract of the adult brain.[26]

Tracts of the DAL lineages are closely associated with the lobes and peduncle of the mushroom body (Fig. 12H); they form a major part of the "circumferential mushroom body systems" of the larval brain (Fig. 11B,D). Most SATs of the DAL lineages pass through and/or terminate in the BC compartment (= ventral body in the adult brain) and the primordium of the central complex (trCM, DPC1; Fig. 12H). A number of tracts cross dorsal of the central complex primordium (DAC3, the future arched commissure of the ventral body) or ventral of it (VAC3/4; sub-ellipsoid commissure/inter ventral body connective). These trajectories support the idea that many of the neurons that innervate the central complex and interconnect this structure with the ventral body are derivatives of the DAL lineages.

Several DAL tracts have ventrally directed branches that follow the central anterior protocerebral tract (CAPT) which is established already in the late embryo.[52,57] We surmise that this connection between brain (i.e., supraesophageal ganglion) and ventral nerve cord (i.e., subesophageal ganglion) will develop into the fiber bundle called subesophageal-ventro-lateral tract in the adult.[26] The contribution of ascending and descending fibers to this fiber system has not been investigated in detail. It seems likely that many of the lateral deuterocerebral descending neurons identified by Strausfeld and collaborators are derivatives of the DAL lineages.[61]

Lineages of the Dorsal Protocerebrum

Two groups of lineages, DPM and DPL, occupy the dorsal surface of the brain. Their axon tracts form the bulk of commissural and longitudinal connections of the dorsal protocerebrum that constitute the DP and CPL compartments (differentiated into superior-medial and inferior-medial protocerebrum, superior-lateral and inferior lateral protocerebrum and lateral horn in the adult brain; Figs. 11B; 12A,I,J; 13C,G,J).[26] The tracts formed by the DPLc and DPLl lineages that penetrate into the protocerebrum in ventro-medial direction are likely the forerunners of the so called "medial and lateral intracerebral cascades" of the adult brain (Fig. 12J).[26] The longitudinally directed fiber masses produced by DPM and DPL lineages, i.e., the loDM and loDL, foreshadow the dorsal horizontal tract and lateral dorsal horizontal tract of the adult protocerebrum (Figs.11B,D; 12I,J).[26] The most conspicuous commissure of the adult dorsal protocerebrum is the commissure of the lateral horn, in addition to a number of unnamed commissural tracts posterior to this system. These fiber systems are likely descended from the DPC2/3 commissures that are formed in the larva by SATs of (among others) the DPM and DPL lineages (Fig. 13H,K).

Lateral Protocerebral Lineages

Lateral protocerebral lineages (BL) have tracts that radially converge towards each other and form the BPL compartment (Figs.11A; 12K; 13A-C). In the larva, the SATs of the BL lineages form the system of external tracts (exBL, exDL, exVT; Figs. 11C, D; 12K). The BPL compartment undergoes enormous growth and diversification during metamorphosis, mainly due to the in-growth of axons from the lobula of the optic lobe (compare BPL in Fig. 13G and J). BL lineage-derived neurons along with the optic lobe afferents form the so called optic foci of the adult brain.[26] The external fiber systems of the larva develop into the longitudinal and vertical connections in between optic foci. Two transverse systems, the trDL and trBL, carry branches of BL SATs. The trBL and its continuation, VPC2, can easily be recognized as the forerunner of the large commissure of the optic foci defined for the adult brain (Fig. 11C,D; 13K).[26] The fate of the trDL, a massive fiber system of the larval dorso-lateral protocerebrum (Fig. 11C), is unclear.

Lineages of the Posterior Protocerebrum

Lineages located at the posterior pole of the brain, including the mushroom body (MB) and CP lineages, project anteriorly and interconnect the dorsal protocerebrum with the deutero-protocerebral boundary region and the deuterocerebrum (Fig. 12A,B,L). The central compartments of the neuropile, CPM, CPI and the mushroom body, arise as cylindrical domains around the axon tracts of these posterior lineages (Figs. 12B; 13A-F). MB lineages give rise to the calyx, peduncle and lobes of the mushroom body whose development has been studied in detail in several recent papers.[27-30,62,63] CP lineages are close to the mushroom body and give rise to two main fiber systems. One is directed anteriorly, parallel to the peduncle and appears to end close to the BC compartment (ventral body). The other crosses over the proximal peduncle and then turns anteriorly and medially towards the primordium of the central complex. While crossing, these axons (the trPd) follow the trajectory that is taken by the commissure of the lateral horn (Figs. 11D; 12L).

Outlook

Adressing fundamental problems of neurobiology in *Drosophila* offers many advantages, as well as some disadvantages. Among the latter is the small size of neurons and the fact that establishing functional relationships between neurons, recordings have to be made from often minuscule neurites within the neuropile, rather than nerve cell somata. Due to these anatomical features (shared among many invertebrate animals) we still know very little about synaptic relationships between neurons in the central nervous system. On the other hand, thanks to the abundance of molecular markers and genetic techniques, it is now possible to map individual cell types of the *Drosophila* nervous system throughout development with an accuracy that is unparalleled in the animal kingdom, with the possible exception of the nematode C. elegans. Recent work summarized in this chapter has started to lay the groundwork to map neurons and their connections relative to discrete landmarks, such as neuropile compartments and lineage tracts. Given sufficient enthusiasm and support from the neurobiological community, the goal of reconstructing neuronal circuitry in its entirety, rather than in a few representative neuronal subsets like the mushroom body, is within reach.

Acknowledgements

This work was supported by NIH Grant RO1 NS29367 to V.H.

References

1. Urbach R, Technau GM. Molecular markers for identified neuroblasts in the developing brain of Drosophila. Development 2003; 130(16):3621-3637.
2. Younossi-Hartenstein A, Nassif C, Green P et al. Early neurogenesis of the Drosophila brain. J Comp Neurol 1996; 370(3):313-329.
3. Hartenstein V, Rudloff E, Campos-Ortega JA. The pattern of proliferation of the neuroblasts in the wild-type embryo of Drosophila melanogaster. Dev Genes Evol 1987; 196:473-485.
4. Brody T, Odenwald WF. Cellular diversity in the developing nervous system: a temporal view from Drosophila. Development 2002; 129(16):3763-3770.
5. Ito K, Hotta Y. Proliferation pattern of postembryonic neuroblasts in the brain of Drosophila melanogaster. Dev Biol 1992; 149(1):134-148.
6. Ceron J, Gonzalez C, Tejedor FJ. Patterns of cell division and expression of asymmetric cell fate determinants in postembryonic neuroblast lineages of Drosophila. Dev Biol 2001; 230(2):125-138.

7. Dumstrei K, Wang F, Hartenstein V. Role of DE-cadherin in neuroblast proliferation, neural morphogenesis and axon tract formation in Drosophila larval brain development. J Neurosci 2003; 23(8):3325-3335.
8. Dumstrei K, Wang F, Nassif C et al. Early development of the Drosophila brain: V. Pattern of postembryonic neuronal lineages expressing DE-cadherin. J Comp Neurol 2003; 455(4):451-462.
9. Rolls MM, Albertson R, Shih HP et al. Drosophila aPKC regulates cell polarity and cell proliferation in neuroblasts and epithelia. J Cell Biol 2003; 163(5):1089-1098.
10. Schaefer M, Shevchenko A, Knoblich JA et al. A protein complex containing Inscuteable and the Galpha-binding protein Pins orients asymmetric cell divisions in Drosophila. Curr Biol 2000; 10(7):353-362.
11. Schober M, Schaefer M, Knoblich JA. Bazooka recruits Inscuteable to orient asymmetric cell divisions in Drosophila neuroblasts. Nature 1999; 402(6761):548-551.
12. Wodarz A, Ramrath A, Kuchinke U et al. Bazooka provides an apical cue for Inscuteable localization in Drosophila neuroblasts. Nature 1999; 402(6761):544-547.
13. Maurange C, Gould AP. Brainy but not too brainy: starting and stopping neuroblast divisions in Drosophila. Trends Neurosci 2005; 28(1):30-36.
14. Isshiki T, Pearson B, Holbrook S et al. Drosophila neuroblasts sequentially express transcription factors which specify the temporal identity of their neuronal progeny. Cell 2001; 106(4):511-521.
15. Bilder D. Cell polarity: squaring the circle. Curr Biol 2001; 11(4):R132-135.
16. Doe CQ, Bowerman B. Asymmetric cell division: fly neuroblast meets worm zygote. Curr Opin Cell Biol 2001; 13(1):68-75.
17. Ebens AJ, Garren H, Cheyette BN et al. The Drosophila anachronism locus: a glycoprotein secreted by glia inhibits neuroblast proliferation. Cell 1993; 74(1):15-27.
18. Bello BC, Hirth F, Gould AP. A pulse of the Drosophila Hox protein Abdominal-A schedules the end of neural proliferation via neuroblast apoptosis. Neuron 2003; 37(2):209-219.
19. Voigt A, Pflanz R, Schafer U et al. Perlecan participates in proliferation activation of quiescent Drosophila neuroblasts. Dev Dyn 2002; 224(4):403-412.
20. Park Y, Rangel C, Reynolds MM et al. Drosophila perlecan modulates FGF and hedgehog signals to activate neural stem cell division. Dev Biol 2003; 253(2):247-257.
21. Datta S. Control of proliferation activation in quiescent neuroblasts of the Drosophila central nervous system. Development 1995; 121(4):1173-1182.
22. Caldwell MC, Datta S. Expression of cyclin E or DP/E2F rescues the G1 arrest of trol mutant neuroblasts in the Drosophila larval central nervous system. Mech Dev 1998; 79(1-2):121-130.
23. Park Y, Ng C, Datta S. Induction of string rescues the neuroblast proliferation defect in trol mutant animals. Genesis 2003; 36(4):187-195.
24. Almeida MS, Bray SJ. Regulation of post-embryonic neuroblasts by Drosophila Grainyhead. Mech Dev 2005; 122(12):1282-1293.
25. Akong K, Grevengoed EE, Price MH et al. Drosophila APC2 and APC1 play overlapping roles in wingless signaling in the embryo and imaginal discs. Dev Biol 2002; 250(1):91-100.
26. Strausfeld NJ. Altas of an Insect Brain. Springer, 1976.
27. Crittenden JR, Skoulakis EM, Han KA et al. Tripartite mushroom body architecture revealed by antigenic markers. Learn Mem 1998; 5(1-2):38-51.
28. Ito K, Awano W, Suzuki K et al. The Drosophila mushroom body is a quadruple structure of clonal units each of which contains a virtually identical set of neurones and glial cells. Development 1997; 124(4):761-771.
29. Noveen A, Daniel A, Hartenstein V. Early development of the Drosophila mushroom body: the roles of eyeless and dachshund. Development 2000; 127(16):3475-3488.
30. Tettamanti M, Armstrong JD, Endo K et al. Early development of the Drosophila mushroom bodies, brain centres for associative learning and memory. Dev Genes Evol 1997; 207(4):242-252.
31. Ito K, Suzuki K, Estes P et al. The organization of extrinsic neurons and their implications in the functional roles of the mushroom bodies in Drosophila melanogaster Meigen. Learn Mem 1998; 5(1-2):52-77.
32. Bossing T, Udolph G, Doe CQ et al. The embryonic central nervous system lineages of Drosophila melanogaster. I. Neuroblast lineages derived from the ventral half of the neuroectoderm. Dev Biol 1996; 179(1):41-64.
33. Schmidt H, Rickert C, Bossing T et al. The embryonic central nervous system lineages of Drosophila melanogaster. II. Neuroblast lineages derived from the dorsal part of the neuroectoderm. Dev Biol 1997; 189(2):186-204.
34. Prokop A, Meinertzhagen IA. Development and structure of synaptic contacts in Drosophila. Semin Cell Dev Biol 2006; 17(1):20-30.

35. Sanchez-Soriano N, Bottenberg W, Fiala A et al. Are dendrites in Drosophila homologous to vertebrate dendrites? Dev Biol 2005; 288(1):126-138.

36. Clark IE, Jan LY, Jan YN. Reciprocal localization of Nod and kinesin fusion proteins indicates microtubule polarity in the Drosophila oocyte, epithelium, neuron and muscle. Development 1997; 124(2):461-470.

37. Chang T, Younossi-Hartenstein A, Hartenstein V. Development of neural lineages derived from the sine oculis positive eye field of Drosophila. Arhtropod Stru Dev 2003; 32:303-317.

38. Pereanu W, Hartenstein V. Neural lineages of the Drosophila brain: a three-dimensional digital atlas of the pattern of lineage location and projection at the late larval stage. J Neurosci 2006; 26(20):5534-5553.

39. Cantera R. Glial cells in adult and developing prothoracic ganglion of the hawk moth Manduca sexta. Cell Tiss Res 1993; 272:93-108.

40. Hoyle G. Glial cells of an insect ganglion. J Comp Neurol 1986; 246(1):85-103.

41. Ito K, Urbach R, Technau GM. Distribution, classification and development of Drosophila glia cells in the late embryonic and early larval ventral nerve cord. Dev Genes Evol 1995; 204:284-307.

42. Saint Marie RL, Carlson SD, Chi C. The Glial Cells of Insects. New York, NY: Plenum 1984.

43. Lane N. Insect intercellular junctions: Their structure and development. New York: Plenum 1982.

44. Hoyle G, Williams M, Phillips C. Functional morphology of insect neuronal cell-surface/glial contacts: the trophospongium. J Comp Neurol 1986; 246(1):113-128.

45. Hidalgo A. Neuron-glia interactions during axon guidance in Drosophila. Biochem Soc Trans 2003; 31(Pt 1):50-55.

46. Pielage J, Klambt C. Glial cells aid axonal target selection. Trends Neurosci 2001; 24(8):432-433.

47. Sepp KJ, Auld VJ. Reciprocal interactions between neurons and glia are required for Drosophila peripheral nervous system development. J Neurosci 2003; 23(23):8221-8230.

48. Sepp KJ, Schulte J, Auld VJ. Peripheral glia direct axon guidance across the CNS/PNS transition zone. Dev Biol 2001; 238(1):47-63.

49. Oland LA, Tolbert LP. Key interactions between neurons and glial cells during neural development in insects. Annu Rev Entomol 2003; 48:89-110.

50. Hartenstein V, Nassif C, Lekven A. Embryonic development of the Drosophila brain. II. Pattern of glial cells. J Comp Neurol 1998; 402(1):32-47.

51. Pereanu W, Shy D, Hartenstein V. Morphogenesis and proliferation of the larval brain glia in Drosophila. Dev Biol 2005; 283(1):191-203.

52. Younossi-Hartenstein A, Nguyen B, Shy D et al. Embryonic origin of the Drosophila brain neuropile. J Comp Neurol 2006; 497(6):981-998.

53. Pereanu W, Spindler S, Cruz L et al. Tracheal development in the Drosophila brain is constrained by glial cells. Dev Biol 2006.

54. Manning G, Krasnow MA. Development of the Drosophila tracheal system. New York: Cold Spring Harbor, Laboratory Press 1993.

55. Englund C, Uv AE, Cantera R et al. adrift, a novel bnl-induced Drosophila gene, required for tracheal pathfinding into the CNS. Development 1999; 126(7):1505-1514.

56. Nassif C, Noveen A, Hartenstein V. Embryonic development of the Drosophila brain. I. Pattern of pioneer tracts. J Comp Neurol 1998; 402(1):10-31.

57. Nassif C, Noveen A, Hartenstein V. Early development of the Drosophila brain: III. The pattern of neuropile founder tracts during the larval period. J Comp Neurol 2003; 455(4):417-434.

58. Goodman CS, Doe CQ. Embryonic development of the Drosophila central nervous system. New York: Cold Spring Harbor Laboratory Press, 1993.

59. Hirth F, Kammermeier L, Frei E et al. An urbilaterian origin of the tripartite brain: developmental genetic insights from Drosophila. Development 2003; 130(11):2365-2373.

60. Therianos S, Leuzinger S, Hirth F et al. Embryonic development of the Drosophila brain: formation of commissural and descending pathways. Development 1995; 121(11):3849-3860.

61. Strausfeld NJ, Bassemir U, Singh RN et al. Organizational principles of outputs from Dipteran brains. J Ins Physiol 1984; 30(1):73-93.

62. Armstrong JD, de Belle JS, Wang Z et al. Metamorphosis of the mushroom bodies; large-scale rearrangements of the neural substrates for associative learning and memory in Drosophila. Learn Mem 1998; 5(1-2):102-114.

63. Zhu S, Chiang AS, Lee T. Development of the Drosophila mushroom bodies: elaboration, remodeling and spatial organization of dendrites in the calyx. Development 2003; 130(12):2603-2610.

Anteroposterior Regionalization of the Brain:
Genetic and Comparative Aspects

Robert Lichtneckert* and Heinrich Reichert

Abstract

Developmental genetic analyses of embryonic CNS development in *Drosophila* have uncovered the role of key, high-order developmental control genes in anteroposterior regionalization of the brain. The gene families that have been characterized include the *otd/Otx* and *ems/Emx* genes which are involved in specification of the anterior brain, the *Hox* genes which are involved in the differentiation of the posterior brain and the *Pax* genes which are involved in the development of the anterior/posterior brain boundary zone. Taken together with work on the genetic control of mammalian CNS development, these findings indicate that all three gene sets have evolutionarily conserved roles in brain development, revealing a surprising evolutionary conservation in the molecular mechanisms of brain regionalization.

Introduction

In most animals, the central nervous system (CNS) is characterized by bilateral symmetry and by an elongated anteroposterior axis, both of which are established very early in embryonic development. During embryogenesis, regionalized anatomical subdivisions appear along the anteroposterior axis, also referred to as the neuraxis. These subdivisions are most prominent near the anterior pole, where the complex structures that comprise the brain are generated. As the brain differentiates, the neuraxis often bends and species-specific flexures arise, which in later stages tend to distort the original anteroposterior coordinates of the CNS. However, when this is taken into account and the neuraxis is reconstructed, remarkable similarities in anteroposterior regionalization of the CNS in animals as diverse as arthropods and vertebrates become apparent. A full appreciation of these similarities comes from combined comparative neuroanatomical and molecular genetic studies carried out in *Drosophila* and mouse, which reveal that comparable, evolutionarily conserved developmental patterning mechanisms operate in regionalization of the embryonic CNS.[1,2]

Here we review recent findings on the developmental genetic control of anteroposterior regionalization in the embryonic CNS in *Drosophila* and compare these findings with investigations carried out on regionalization of the embryonic murine CNS. The similarities in the expression patterns of key developmental control genes together with the comparable functions of these genes during CNS development in flies and mice suggest a common evolutionary origin of the mechanism of embryonic CNS regionalization. Given the current molecular-based phylogeny of bilaterian animals, it seems likely that these features of brain development in arthropods and vertebrates were already present in the common bilaterian ancestor from which protostomes and deuterostomes evolved (Fig. 1).[3] This, in turn, challenges the classical view of an independent origin of protostome and deuterostome brains.

*Corresponding Author: Robert Lichtneckert—Biozentrum, University of Basel, Klingelbergstrasse 50, CH-4056 Basel, Switzerland. Email: robert.lichtneckert@stud.unibas.ch

Brain Development in Drosophila melanogaster, edited by Gerhard M. Technau.
©2008 Landes Bioscience and Springer Science+Business Media.

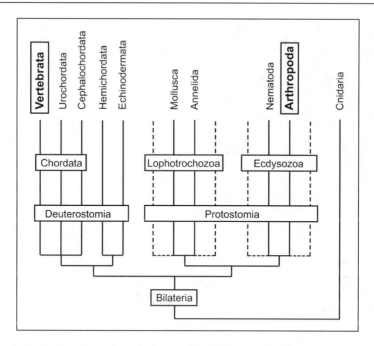

Figure 1. Phylogenetic relationship of Bilateria. Simplified version of the new molecular-based phylogeny showing a selection of bilaterian phyla with the Cnidaria as outgroup. Bilaterian phyla are grouped according to major cladistic classifications. The phylogenetic tree suggests that evolutionarily conserved, homologous features of mouse and *D. melanogaster* already existed in the common ancestor of all bilaterian animals.

The early embryonic CNS of both insects and vertebrates is composed of longitudinally arranged subdivisions that can be grouped into two major parts, an anterior cephalized brain which rapidly forms prominent morphological specializations and a posterior nerve cord-like structure. In insects, the embryonic brain consists of a supraesophageal ganglion that can be subdivided into the protocerebral (b1), deutocerebral (b2) and tritocerebral (b3) neuromeres and a subesophageal ganglion that is subdivided into the mandibular (s1), maxillary (s2) and labial (s3) neuromeres (Fig. 2A). The neuromeres of the developing ventral nerve cord extend posteriorly from the subesophageal ganglion into the body trunk.[4] In vertebrates, the anterior CNS develops three embryological brain regions; the prosencephalon or forebrain (presumptive telencephalon and diencephalon), the mesencephalon or midbrain and the rhombencephalon or hindbrain. The developing hindbrain reveals a metameric organization based on eight rhombomeres and parts of the developing forebrain may also be metamerically organized.[5,6] The developing spinal cord extends posteriorly from the hindbrain into the body trunk.

The topology of these embryonic neuroanatomical regions is reflected in the regionalized expression along the neuraxis of key developmental control genes which appears to be largely conserved between insects and vertebrates. Thus, the anterior CNS of *Drosophila* and mouse is characterized by the expression of the genes *orthodenticle* (*otd/Otx*) and *empty spiracles* (*ems/Emx*). Similarly, the posterior CNS of both species exhibits a conserved and highly ordered expression pattern of the homeotic (*Hox*) gene family. Finally, expression of the *Pax2/5/8* genes defines a third CNS region between the anterior *otd/Otx* and the posterior *Hox* domains, thus revealing a tripartite ground plan of embryonic CNS development in both vertebrates and insects. In the following we consider the roles of each of these three sets of developmental control genes in anteroposterior regionalization of the CNS.

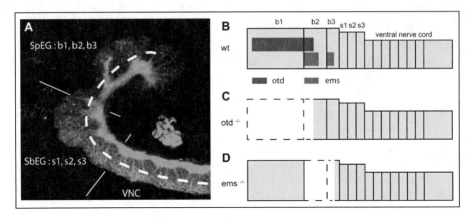

Figure 2. Schematic representation of expression patterns and mutant phenotypes of *otd* and *ems* in the embryonic CNS of *Drosophila*. A) Lateral view of the anterior portion of the embryonic CNS. Because of morphogenetic processes, such as the beginning of head involution, the neuraxis (dashed line) of the embryonic brain curves dorsoposteriorly withing the embryo. Accordingly, in the following, anteroposterior coordinates refer to the neuraxis rather than the embryonic body axis. The major anteroposterior CNS regions are subdivided by white lines. B-D) Schematic representations of the embryonic brain with anterior towards the left and posterior towards the right. B) In the wild type (wt) brain the *otd* gene is expressed throughout most of the protocerebrum (b1) and the anterior part of the deutocerebrum (b2). Expression of *ems* in the brain is restricted to the anterior part of the deutocerebrum and the anterior part of the tritocerebrum (b3). The segmentally reiterated expression patterns of both *otd* and *ems* are omitted for clarity in this schematic. C) In *otd* mutant embryos (*otd*⁻/⁻) the protocerebrum and the anterior deutocerebrum are absent (indicated by dashed lines). D) Mutational inactivation of *ems* (*ems*⁻/⁻) results in the absence of the deutocerebrum and anterior part of the tritocerebrum. Abbreviations: b1, protocerebrum; b2, deutocerebrum; b3, tritocerebrum; s1, mandibular neuromere; s2, maxillary neuromere; s3, labial neuromere; SbEG, subesophageal ganglion; SpEG, supraesophageal ganglion; VNC, ventral nerve cord.

The Cephalic Gap Genes *Otd/Otx* and *Ems/Emx*
Control Anterior Brain Development

The *orthodenticle* (*otd*) and *empty spiracles* (*ems*) homeobox genes belong to the cephalic gap genes in *Drosophila* together with *tailless* (*tll*), *buttonhead* (*btd*) and *sloppy paired* (*slp*). At the early blastoderm stage of embryogenesis, the cephalic gap genes are broadly expressed in overlapping anterior domains under the control of maternal genes.[7-9] The functional inactivation of any of these transcription factors results in gap-like phenotypes where structures of several head segments are missing.[10,11] In addition, the cephalic gap genes *tll*, *otd*, *ems* and *btd* have been shown to play essential roles in early brain development. By the time of neuroblast delamination, their expression domains become restricted to specific subsets of neural progenitors in the anterior procephalic neuroectoderm.[12,13] Mutational inactivation of a given cephalic gap gene results in the deletion of a specific brain area, indicating the requirement of these genes in early specification of the anterior brain primordium.[13,14]

The cephalic gap gene *otd* encodes a transcription factor with a *bicoid*-like homeodomain and is required for head development and segmental patterning in the fly embryo. In the early blastoderm stage embryo, *otd* is first expressed in a broad circumferential stripe in the anterior region. During gastrulation, however, expression becomes more and more restricted to the anterior procephalic neuroectoderm, where *otd* is expressed in most delaminating neuroblasts of the presumptive protocerebrum (b1) and anterior deutocerebrum (b2).[12,13] This expression domain corresponds largely to the *otd* expression pattern detected at later embryonic stages in the brain[14]

(Fig. 2B). Interestingly, *otd* expression is not observed in the anterior most protocerebral region. An additional, segmentally reiterated expression pattern of *otd* is found at the ventral midline of the fly embryo in mesectodermal cells that will give rise to neurons and glia of the ventral nerve cord (not shown in Fig. 2B). Comparable to *otd*, the homeobox gene *ems* is first expressed in a broad stripe posterior and adjacent to *otd* in the early blastoderm stage embryo. In the procephalic neuroectoderm and in the subsequently formed early embryonic brain *ems* expression becomes restricted to two stripes in the anterior parts of the deutocerebral (b2) and tritocerebral (b3) neuromeres (Fig. 2B). In the ventral nerve cord *ems* expression is also found in a segmentally repeated pattern (not shown in Fig. 2B).[14,15]

Mutational inactivation of either *otd* or *ems* results in striking embryonic brain phenotypes in which large brain regions are absent. In the *otd* mutant the entire anterior part of the brain is lacking (Fig. 2C) and mutant analysis has shown that most protocerebral neuroblasts and part of the adjacent deutocerebral neuroblasts are absent in the procephalic neuroectoderm.[13,14] In addition to the gap phenotype in the anterior brain, *otd* mutant flies exhibit impairments in the development of visual structures as well as midline defects in the ventral nerve cord.[8] Ubiquitous overexpression of *otd* in a null mutant background at specific stages preceding neuroblast formation is able to restore anterior brain structures and ventral nerve cord defects.[16] Similarly, loss-of-function of the *ems* gene results in a gap-like phenotype in the embryonic brain due to the absence of cells in the deutocerebral and tritocerebral neuromeres (Fig. 2D). Additionally, axon pathfinding defects can be observed in the ventral nerve cord of *ems* mutant embryos. These phenotypes are rescued by ubiquitous overexpression of *ems* during specific early embryonic stages.[15] Mutant analysis for both *otd* and *ems* shows that the absence of cephalic gap gene expression in the procephalic neuroectoderm correlates with the loss in the expression of the proneural gene *lethal of scute* (*l'sc*) and the ability to form neuroblasts in the mutant domain.[13] In summary, *otd* and *ems* are expressed in adjacent and slightly overlapping domains in the anterior embryonic fly brain. The function of these cephalic gap genes is required for the formation of specific regions of the anterior brain primordium.

Based on homology between homeobox sequences, orthologs of the *Drosophila otd* and *ems* genes have been isolated in various vertebrates including zebrafish, mouse and humans.[17,18] In mouse, the two vertebrate orthologs of the *otd* gene, *Otx1* and *Otx,2* are expressed in nested domains of the developing head and brain. *Otx1* transcripts first appear at approximately 8 days post coitum (dpc), whereas *Otx2* expression is detectable earlier at the prestreak stage (5.5 dpc) within the entire epiblast and visceral endoderm prior to the onset of gastrulation. Subsequently, the domain of *Otx2* expression becomes restricted to the anterior region of the embryo, which includes a territory fated to give rise to forebrain and midbrain, defining a sharp boundary at the future midbrain-hindbrain boundary. *Otx1* expression is nested within this *Otx2* domain and subsequently becomes spatially and temporally restricted to the developing cortex and cerebellum. Interestingly, the domain of *Otx2* expression does not include the most anterior brain region, which is similar to the expression pattern of *otd* in the embryonic fly brain.[17,19] Analysis of *Otx1* mutants does not reveal any apparent defects in early brain development. However, later in development loss of *Otx1* function affects cortical neurogenesis and causes epilepsy. In addition, the development of eye and inner ear is impaired.[17,20] In contrast to *Otx1* mutant mice, *Otx2* null mice die early in embryogenesis and lack the rostral brain regions including forebrain, midbrain and rostral hindbrain due to defective anterior neuroectoderm specification.[17, 21]

A comparison of the role of the *otd*/*Otx* genes in early brain patterning in *Drosophila* and mouse reveals striking similarities suggesting an evolutionary conservation of *otd*/*Otx* gene function. An interesting confirmation of the functional conservation in patterning the rostral brain can be carried out in cross-phylum rescue experiments. Ubiquitous overexpression of either human *Otx1* or human *Otx2* in an *otd* mutant fly embryo restores the anterior brain structures absent in the *otd* null mutant.[16] Similarly, overexpression of *Drosophila otd* in an *Otx1* null mouse embryo fully rescues epilepsy and corticogenesis abnormalities (but not inner ear defects).[17,22] Moreover, overexpression of a hybrid transcript consisting of the fly *otd* coding region fused to the 5' and

3' UTRs of *Otx2* restores the anterior brain patterning in *Otx2* null mutant mice including the normal positioning of the midbrain-hindbrain boundary.[23]

As is the case for the *otd*/*Otx* genes, two vertebrate orthologs of the *Drosophila ems* gene, *Emx1* and *Emx2*, have been identified. *Emx1* and *Emx2* expression in the mouse CNS is restricted to the forebrain, where largely overlapping expression patterns are seen. Whereas, *Emx1* expression only begins after neurulation, *Emx2* is already detectable around 8.5 dpc in the rostral neural plate.[19,24,25] Within the developing neocortex, *Emx2* is expressed in a high caudomedial to low rostrolateral gradient, which is contrasted by an opposed gradient of *Pax6* gene expression. Mutational inactivation of *Emx2* results in an expansion of the rostrolateral brain areas at the expense of the caudomedial neocortical areas. An opposite shift in regional identity is seen in the *Pax6* loss-of-function mutant. In the *Emx2* and *Pax6* double mutant, the cerebral cortex completely loses its identity and instead acquires characteristics of basal ganglia.[26,27] Whereas *Emx2* mutant mice die immediately after birth, *Emx1* mutant animals are postnatal viable and show rather subtle phenotypes that are restricted to the forebrain.[28,29] The regionalized expression patterns of the *ems*/*Emx* genes in the developing brain of *Drosophila* and mouse are remarkably similar, as is their ability to confer regional identity to the cells of a specific domain in the brain. Moreover, overexpression of a mouse *Emx2* transgene in an *ems* mutant background can rescue the brain phenotype of fly embryos.[15] Taken together, the similar spatiotemporal expression patterns and the high degree of functional equivalence between *Drosophila* and mouse suggest an evolutionarily conserved role of the *ems*/*Emx* and *otd*/*Otx* genes in anterior brain development.

The *Hox* Genes Pattern the Posterior Brain

The homeotic or *Hox* genes, encoding homeodomain transcription factors, were first discovered as crucial regulators of anteroposterior segment identity in the ectoderm of *Drosophila melanogaster*. Subsequently, *Hox* genes were found in a wide range of species where they have essential roles in many aspects of anteroposterior body axis patterning.[30,31] In *Drosophila*, the *Hox* genes are arranged along the chromosome in two gene clusters known as the *Antennapedia* (*ANT-C*) and *Bithorax* (*BX-C*) complexes. The *ANT-C* contains the five more anteriorly expressed *Hox* genes: *labial* (*lab*), *proboscipedia* (*pb*), *Deformed* (*Dfd*), *Sex combs reduced* (*Scr*) and *Antennapedia* (*Antp*). The *BX-C* contains the three posteriorly expressed genes: *Ultrabithorax* (*Ubx*), *abdominal-A* (*abd-A*) and *Abdominal-B* (*Abd-B*). Interestingly, there exists a correlation between the relative position of the genes within the cluster and their spatial and temporal expression pattern along the body axis; genes located towards the 3' end of the cluster are expressed more anteriorly and earlier in the embryo than are genes located towards the 5' end. This correlation has been termed spatial and temporal colinearity.[32] In mammals, *Hox* genes are arranged into four chromosomal clusters, termed *Hox A–D*, which contain between 9 and 11 *Hox* genes that can be assigned to 13 paralogous groups. Only the *Hox B* cluster comprises orthologs of all *Drosophila* homeotic genes. As in *Drosophila*, spatial and temporal colinearity is also observed among vertebrate *Hox* genes and more posterior acting genes impose their developmental specificities upon anterior acting genes.[32,33]

Hox gene expression in the developing CNS is a shared feature of a wide range of bilaterian animals, including protostomes such as insects or annelids and deuterostomes, such as hemichordates or vertebrates.[34-37] Remarkably, throughout the Bilateria, *Hox* gene orthologs are expressed in a similar anteroposterior order. In *Drosophila*, the expressions of *Hox* cluster genes delineate discrete domains in the embryonic brain and ventral nerve cord (Fig. 3A). Their anterior expression boundaries often coincide with morphologically defined neuromere compartment boundaries. Although the anteroposterior order of *Hox* gene expression domains largely follows the spatial colinearity rule known from ectodermal structures, one important difference is noteworthy: expression of the two 3'-most *Hox* genes of the *ANT-C* is inverted, in that the anterior expression boundary of *lab* lies posterior to that of *pb*.[34] Interestingly, this particularity of the *Hox* expression pattern in the CNS is common to fly and mouse. In vertebrates, *Hox* genes are expressed in the developing hindbrain and spinal cord. The relative anteroposterior order of *Hox* gene expression in the CNS of vertebrates is virtually identical to their arrangement in *Drosophila*, including the inverted order of the *lab* and *pb* orthologs, *Hoxb-1* and *Hoxb-2* (Fig. 3B).[38] As more expression data from different protostome and deuterostome species becomes available, the ordered expression of *Hox* genes along the anteroposterior axis of the developing nervous system is likely to consolidate as a common feature of bilaterian animals.

In *Drosophila*, mutational inactivation of either of the homeotic genes *lab* or *Dfd* causes severe axonal patterning defects in the embryonic brain.[34] In *lab* null mutants, axonal projection defects are observed in the posterior tritocerebrum where *lab* is expressed in the wild type brain. In the mutant, longitudinal pathways connecting supraesophageal and subesophageal ganglia as well as projections in the tritocerebral commissure are absent or reduced. These brain defects are not due to deletions in the affected neuromere; neuronal progenitors are present and give rise to progeny in the mutant domain. However, these postmitotic progeny fail to acquire a neuronal identity, as indicated by the absence of neuronal markers and the lack of axonal and dendritic extensions (Fig. 3A). Comparable defects are seen in *Dfd* mutants in the corresponding mandibular/anterior maxillary domain, where the gene is expressed in the wild type brain.[34] Thus, the activity of the homeotic genes *lab* and *Dfd* is necessary to establish regionalized neuronal identity in the brain of *Drosophila*.

The mouse *lab* orthologs, *Hoxa-1* and *Hoxb-1*, are expressed in overlapping domains with a sharp anterior boundary coinciding with the presumptive rhombomere 3/4 border. Functional inactivation of *Hoxa-1* results in segmentation defects leading to a reduced size of rhombomeres 4 and 5 and defects in motor neuron axonal projections but the normal identity of rhombomere 4 is not altered.[39] In contrast, loss of *Hoxb-1* function has no influence on the size of rhombomere 4 but causes a partial transformation into a rhombomere 2 identity.[40] The *Hoxa-1, Hoxb-1* double mutant results in a territory of unknown identity and reduced size between rhombomeres 3 and 5, suggesting a synergistic action of the two genes in rhombomere 4 specification (Fig. 3B).[39] Thus, the concerted activity of *Hoxa-1* and *Hoxb-1* has a similar role in the specification of the regionalized neuronal identity as does their ortholog *lab* in the CNS of *Drosophila*. This suggests a functional conservation of *Hox* genes, in addition to a similar mode of expression, during nervous system development of bilaterian animals and supports the idea of a common origin of the CNS.

Evidence for a Tripartite Organization of the Brain

Comparative gene expression studies, as reviewed here for *Drosophila* and mouse, have been carried out in numerous protostome and deuterostome phyla.[36,41-44] The subdivision of the developing brain into an anterior region specified by genes of the *otd/Otx* family and a posterior region specified by genes of the *Hox* family appears to be a universal feature of bilaterian animals. In vertebrates and urochordates, a third embryonic domain along the anteroposterior neuraxis, characterized by overlapping expression of the *Pax2*, *Pax5* and *Pax8* genes, is located between the anterior *Otx* and the posterior *Hox* expressing regions of the embryonic brain.[45-47] In vertebrate brain development, this *Pax2/5/8* domain is located between the presumptive mesencephalon and metencephalon, where it plays a crucial role in development of the midbrain-hindbrain boundary (MHB) region or isthmus. Transplantation experiments, in which MHB tissue grafts are inserted to more rostral or caudal brain regions inducing ectopic mesencephalic-metencephalic structures, reveal an organizer function of the MHB. This organizer activity on the surrounding neural tissue is thought to be mediated by fibroblast growth factor 8 (Fgf8) and Wnt1 proteins, which are secreted by cells located in the MHB.[45,47] In early embryonic development of the vertebrate CNS, the homeobox gene *Gbx2* is expressed in the anterior hindbrain just posterior to the *Otx2* domain in the forebrain and midbrain. During gastrulation and early neurulation the MHB is established at the *Otx2/Gbx2* interface, where subsequently the expression domains of other MHB markers including *Pax2/5/8*, Fgf8, Wnt1 and *En1/2* are positioned (Fig. 4C). The two homeobox genes *Otx2* and *Gbx2* mutually repress one another and upregulation or downregulation of either gene shifts the position of the MHB accordingly.[45,47] Therefore, in vertebrates an antagonistic interaction between *Otx2* and *Gbx2* during early embryonic development is involved in the correct positioning of the MHB at their common interface.

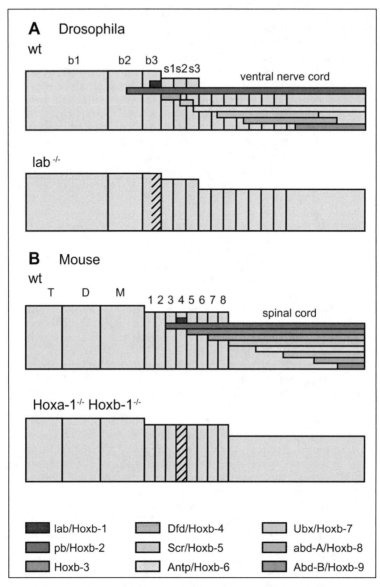

Figure 3. Simplified schematic comparison of *Hox* gene expression domains and mutant phenotypes in the CNS of *Drosophila* and mouse. Schematic representations of the embryonic
brain with anterior towards the left and posterior towards the right. A) Expression domains of
the homeotic genes of the Antennapedia and Bithorax complexes in the CNS of *Drosophila*
(see text for gene nomenclature). In *lab* null mutant embryos (*lab⁻/⁻*), cells of the posterior part
of the tritocerebrum (b3) are correctly located in the mutant domain, but fail to assume their
correct neuronal cell fate (dashed lines). B) Expression of the *Hox* genes *Hoxb-1* to *Hoxb-9* in
the developing mouse CNS. *Hoxa-1⁻/⁻* and *Hoxb-1⁻/⁻* double mutant embryos (*Hoxa-1⁻/⁻*; *Hoxb-1⁻/⁻*)
lose rhombomere 4 identity (dashed lines). Abbreviations: T, telencephalon; D, diencephalon;
M, mesencephalon; 1-8, rhombomeres 1-8; (for other abbreviations see Fig. 2). Modified and
reprinted with permission from: Hirth F et al. Development 1998; 125: 1579-1589. © The
Company of Biologists Limited.

Gene expression studies indicate that a similar tripartite ground plan for anteroposterior regionalization of the embryonic brain is also present in *Drosophila*. The *Drosophila* genome contains two genes, *Pox neuro* (*Poxn*) and *Pax2*, which are together considered to be orthologs of the *Pax2/5/8* genes.[48] Remarkably, expression of both orthologs is present at the interface of *otd* and the *Drosophila Gbx2* ortholog *unplugged* (*unpg*), anterior to a *Hox*-expressing region (Fig. 4A,B).[44] Although *Poxn* and *Pax2* are expressed in a segmentally reiterated pattern along the entire embryonic CNS, their expression at the *otd/unpg* interface is exceptional in two ways. The two genes are expressed in adjacent domains delineating together a transversal stripe of the brain and this is the only position along the neuraxis where expression of both genes coincides with a brain neuromere boundary, the deutocerebral-tritocerebral boundary (DTB) (Fig. 4A,B).[44] Analyses of either *otd* or *unpg* mutants reveal a mutually repressive function of the two genes during early brain patterning. Thus, in *otd* mutant embryos a rostral extension of the *unpg* expression domain is observed (in addition to the deletion of the anterior brain). On the other hand, mutational inactivation of the *unpg* gene results in a caudal shift of the posterior limit of *otd* expression.[44] Therefore, in both *Drosophila* and mouse, the early interaction of *otd/Otx2* and *unpg/Gbx2* is essential for the correct positioning of an intermediate brain domain characterized by a sharply delimited *otd/Otx2* and *unpg/Gbx2* interface and the expression of *Pax2/5/8* genes. In contrast to vertebrates, mutational inactivation of the *Drosophila Pax2/5/8* orthologs *Poxn* or *Pax2* does not appear to result in brain patterning defects. Moreover, to date, there is no evidence of an organizer activity at the fly DTB, suggesting that the organizer function at the *otd/Otx2* and *unpg/Gbx2*

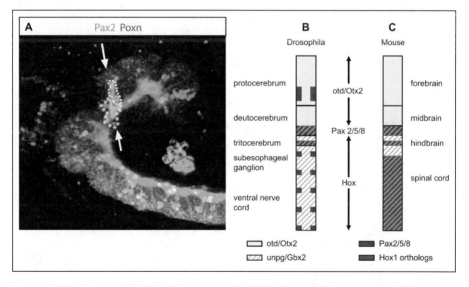

Figure 4. Tripartite organization of the embryonic CNS in *Drosophila* and mouse. A) Expression of *Pax2* and *Poxn* in the brain of stage 13/14 embryos. At the deutocerebral-tritocerebral boundary (indicated by white arrows), *Pax2* (white dots) and *Poxn* (white asterisks) are expressed in adjacent domains forming a transversal line in the CNS (immunolabelled with antiHRP and shown in grey). B,C) The expression of *otd/Otx2*, *unpg/Gbx2*, *Pax2/5/8* and *Hox1* gene orthologs in the developing CNS of *Drosophila* (B) and mouse (C). (In this schematic, anterior is towards the top and posterior is towards the bottom.) In both cases, *otd/Otx2* is expressed in the anterior nervous system rostral to a *Hox*-expressing region in the posterior nervous system. In addition, a *Pax2/5/8*-expressing domain positioned at the interface between the anterior *otd/Otx2* domain and the posteriorly abutting *unpg/Gbx2* expression domain is common to both nervous systems. Modified and reprinted with permission from: Hirth F et al. Development 2003; 130: 2365-2373. © The Company of Biologists Limited.

interface might have emerged after the protostome/deuterostome divergence that separated insects and vertebrates. In fact, an organizer activity of the MHB region has so far only been demonstrated for vertebrate species within deuterostomes.

In summary, current comparative data indicates that similar genetic patterning mechanisms act in anteroposterior regionalization of the developing brain in *Drosophila* and vertebrate species and establish a common, evolutionarily conserved tripartite ground plan. This suggests that a corresponding tripartite organization of the developing brain was already present in the last common bilateral ancestor of insects and vertebrates.

References

1. Arendt D, Nubler-Jung K. Comparison of early nerve cord development in insects and vertebrates. Development 1999; 126(11):2309-2325.
2. Reichert H, Simeone A. Conserved usage of gap and homeotic genes in patterning the CNS. Curr Opin Neurobiol 1999; 9(5):589-595.
3. Adoutte A, Balavoine G, Lartillot N et al. The new animal phylogeny: reliability and implications. Proc Natl Acad Sci USA 2000; 97(9):4453-4456.
4. Younossi-Hartenstein A, Nassif C, Green P et al. Early neurogenesis of the Drosophila brain. J Comp Neurol 1996; 370(3):313-329.
5. Lumsden A, Krumlauf R. Patterning the vertebrate neuraxis. Science 1996; 274(5290):1109-1115.
6. Puelles L, Rubenstein JL. Forebrain gene expression domains and the evolving prosomeric model. Trends Neurosci 2003; 26(9):469-476.
7. Dalton D, Chadwick R, McGinnis W. Expression and embryonic function of empty spiracles: a Drosophila homeo box gene with two patterning functions on the anterior-posterior axis of the embryo. Genes Dev 1989; 3(12A):1940-1956.
8. Finkelstein R, Perrimon N. The orthodenticle gene is regulated by bicoid and torso and specifies Drosophila head development. Nature 1990; 346(6283):485-488.
9. Walldorf U, Gehring WJ. Empty spiracles, a gap gene containing a homeobox involved in Drosophila head development. EMBO J 1992; 11(6):2247-2259.
10. Cohen SM, Jurgens G. Mediation of Drosophila head development by gap-like segmentation genes. Nature 1990; 346(6283):482-485.
11. Schmidt-Ott U, Gonzalez-Gaitan M, Jackle H et al. Number, identity and sequence of the Drosophila head segments as revealed by neural elements and their deletion patterns in mutants. Proc Natl Acad Sci USA 1994; 91(18):8363-8367.
12. Urbach R, Technau GM. Molecular markers for identified neuroblasts in the developing brain of Drosophila. Development 2003; 130(16):3621-3637.
13. Younossi-Hartenstein A, Green P, Liaw GJ et al. Control of early neurogenesis of the Drosophila brain by the head gap genes tll, otd, ems and btd. Dev Biol 1997; 182(2):270-283.
14. Hirth F, Therianos S, Loop T et al. Developmental defects in brain segmentation caused by mutations of the homeobox genes orthodenticle and empty spiracles in Drosophila. Neuron 1995; 15(4):769-778.
15. Hartmann B, Hirth F, Walldorf U et al. Expression, regulation and function of the homeobox gene empty spiracles in brain and ventral nerve cord development of Drosophila. Mech Dev 2000; 90(2):143-153.
16. Leuzinger S, Hirth F, Gerlich D et al. Equivalence of the fly orthodenticle gene and the human OTX genes in embryonic brain development of Drosophila. Development 1998; 125(9):1703-1710.
17. Acampora D, Annino A, Tuorto F et al. Otx genes in the evolution of the vertebrate brain. Brain Res Bull 2005; 66(4-6):410-420.
18. Cecchi C. Emx:2 a gene responsible for cortical development, regionalization and area specification. Gene 2002; 291(1-2):1-9.
19. Simeone A, Acampora D, Gulisano M et al. Nested expression domains of four homeobox genes in developing rostral brain. Nature 1992; 358(6388):687-690.
20. Acampora D, Mazan S, Avantaggiato V et al. Epilepsy and brain abnormalities in mice lacking the Otx1 gene. Nat Genet 1996; 14(2):218-222.
21. Acampora D, Mazan S, Lallemand Y et al. Forebrain and midbrain regions are deleted in Otx2-/- mutants due to a defective anterior neuroectoderm specification during gastrulation. Development 1995; 121(10):3279-3290.
22. Acampora D, Avantaggiato V, Tuorto F et al. Murine Otx1 and Drosophila otd genes share conserved genetic functions required in invertebrate and vertebrate brain development. Development 1998; 125(9):1691-1702.

23. Acampora D, Boyl PP, Signore M et al. OTD/OTX2 functional equivalence depends on 5' and 3' UTR-mediated control of Otx2 mRNA for nucleo-cytoplasmic export and epiblast-restricted translation. Development 2001; 128(23):4801-4813.
24. Simeone A, Gulisano M, Acampora D et al. Two vertebrate homeobox genes related to the Drosophila empty spiracles gene are expressed in the embryonic cerebral cortex. EMBO J 1992; 11(7):2541-2550.
25. Gulisano M, Broccoli V, Pardini C et al. Emx1 and Emx2 show different patterns of expression during proliferation and differentiation of the developing cerebral cortex in the mouse. Eur J Neurosci 1996; 8(5):1037-1050.
26. Bishop KM, Rubenstein JL, O'Leary DD. Distinct actions of Emx1, Emx2 and Pax6 in regulating the specification of areas in the developing neocortex. J Neurosci 1 2002; 22(17):7627-7638.
27. Muzio L, DiBenedetto B, Stoykova A et al. Conversion of cerebral cortex into basal ganglia in Emx2(-/-) Pax6(Sey/Sey) double-mutant mice. Nat Neurosci 2002; 5(8):737-745.
28. Qiu M, Anderson S, Chen S et al. Mutation of the Emx-1 homeobox gene disrupts the corpus callosum. Dev Biol 1996; 178(1):174-178.
29. Yoshida M, Suda Y, Matsuo I et al. Emx1 and Emx2 functions in development of dorsal telencephalon. Development 1997; 124(1):101-111.
30. Ferrier DE, Holland PW. Ancient origin of the Hox gene cluster. Nat Rev Genet 2001; 2(1):33-38.
31. Hughes CL, Kaufman TC. Hox genes and the evolution of the arthropod body plan. Evol Dev 2002; 4(6):459-499.
32. Mann RS. Why are Hox genes clustered? Bioessays 1997; 19(8):661-664.
33. Duboule D, Morata G. Colinearity and functional hierarchy among genes of the homeotic complexes. Trends Genet 1994; 10(10):358-364.
34. Hirth F, Hartmann B, Reichert H. Homeotic gene action in embryonic brain development of Drosophila. Development 1998; 125(9):1579-1589.
35. Kourakis MJ, Master VA, Lokhorst DK et al. Conserved anterior boundaries of Hox gene expression in the central nervous system of the leech Helobdella. Dev Biol 1997; 190(2):284-300.
36. Lowe CJ, Wu M, Salic A et al. Anteroposterior patterning in hemichordates and the origins of the chordate nervous system. Cell 2003; 113(7):853-865.
37. Wilkinson DG, Bhatt S, Cook M et al. Segmental expression of Hox-2 homoeobox-containing genes in the developing mouse hindbrain. Nature 1989; 341(6241):405-409.
38. Hunt P, Krumlauf R. Deciphering the Hox code: clues to patterning branchial regions of the head. Cell 1991; 66(6):1075-1078.
39. Gavalas A, Studer M, Lumsden A et al. Hoxa1 and Hoxb1 synergize in patterning the hindbrain, cranial nerves and second pharyngeal arch. Development 1998; 125(6):1123-1136.
40. Studer M, Lumsden A, Ariza-McNaughton L et al. Altered segmental identity and abnormal migration of motor neurons in mice lacking Hoxb-1. Nature 1996; 384(6610):630-634.
41. Bruce AE, Shankland M. Expression of the head gene Lox22-Otx in the leech Helobdella and the origin of the bilaterian body plan. Dev Biol 1998; 201(1):101-112.
42. Canestro C, Bassham S, Postlethwait J. Development of the central nervous system in the larvacean Oikopleura dioica and the evolution of the chordate brain. Dev Biol 2005; 285(2):298-315.
43. Castro LF, Rasmussen SL, Holland PW et al. A Gbx homeobox gene in amphioxus: Insights into ancestry of the ANTP class and evolution of the midbrain/hindbrain boundary. Dev Biol 2006.
44. Hirth F, Kammermeier L, Frei E et al. An urbilaterian origin of the tripartite brain: developmental genetic insights from Drosophila. Development 2003; 130(11):2365-2373.
45. Liu A, Joyner AL. Early anterior/posterior patterning of the midbrain and cerebellum. Annu Rev Neurosci 2001; 24:869-896.
46. Wada H, Saiga H, Satoh N et al. Tripartite organization of the ancestral chordate brain and the antiquity of placodes: insights from ascidian Pax-2/5/8, Hox and Otx genes. Development 1998; 125(6):1113-1122.
47. Wurst W, Bally-Cuif L. Neural plate patterning: upstream and downstream of the isthmic organizer. Nat Rev Neurosci 2001; 2(2):99-108.
48. Noll M. Evolution and role of Pax genes. Curr Opin Genet Dev 1993; 3(4):595-605.

CHAPTER 3

Dorsoventral Patterning of the Brain:
A Comparative Approach

Rolf Urbach* and Gerhard M. Technau

Abstract

Development of the central nervous system (CNS) involves the transformation of a two-dimensional epithelial sheet of uniform ectodermal cells, the neuroectoderm, into a highly complex three-dimensional structure consisting of a huge variety of different neural cell types. Characteristic numbers of each cell type become arranged in reproducible spatial patterns, which is a prerequisite for the establishment of specific functional contacts. Specification of cell fate and regional patterning critical depends on positional information conferred to neural stem cells early in the neuroectoderm. This chapter compares recent findings on mechanisms that control the specification of cell fates along the dorsoventral axis during embryonic development of the CNS in *Drosophila* and vertebrates. Despite the clear structural differences in the organization of the CNS in arthropods and vertebrates, corresponding domains within the developing brain and truncal nervous system express a conserved set of columnar genes (*msh/Msx, ind/Gsh, vnd/Nkx*) involved in dorsoventral regionalization. In both *Drosophila* and mouse the expression of these genes exhibits distinct differences between the cephalic and truncal part of the CNS. Remarkably, not only the expression of columnar genes shows striking parallels between both species, but to some extent also their genetic interactions, suggesting an evolutionary conservation of key regulators of dorsoventral patterning in the brain in terms of expression and function.

Introduction

The central nervous system (CNS) in *Drosophila* and in vertebrates can be subdivided into two main portions, a truncal part (ventral nerve cord (VNC) in *Drosophila* and spinal cord in vertebrates) composed of repetitive segmental units and an anterior part, the brain, exhibiting a less overt segmental composition (Fig. 1).

In *Drosophila*, the CNS develops from a bilaterally symmetrical sheet of neuroectodermal cells on the ventral side of the embryo. It gives rise to a fixed number of neural stem cells, called neuroblasts (NBs), which segregate to the interior of the embryo. NBs which form the VNC and brain descend from the truncal and procephalic neuroectoderm, respectively (Fig. 2).[1,2] In vertebrates, the CNS forms from a bilaterally symmetrical neuroectoderm on the dorsal side of the embryo. The whole neuroectodermal sheet invaginates to form the neural tube, which develops into the spinal cord and brain. Accordingly, the differentiating NBs do not delaminate but maintain contact with the epithelial surfaces (for a review see ref. 3). Insect and vertebrate NBs divide reiteratively to give rise to specific types of neurons (motoneurons, interneurons) and glial cells.

In *Drosophila*, the border between neurogenic and nonneurogenic ectoderm becomes defined by two antagonistically acting extracellular factors encoded by *short gastrulation* (*sog*) and *decapentaplegic* (*dpp*). The homologous genes in *Xenopus* (vertebrates), *Chordin* and *Bone morphogenetic*

*Corresponding Author: Rolf Urbach—Institute of Genetics, University of Mainz, D-55099 Mainz, Germany. Email: urbach@uni-mainz.de

Brain Development in Drosophila melanogaster, edited by Gerhard M. Technau.
©2008 Landes Bioscience and Springer Science+Business Media.

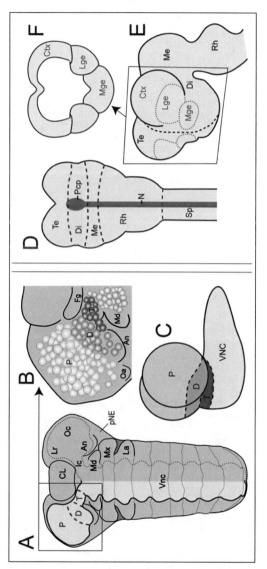

Figure 1. Schematic representations of the morphology and subdivision of the embryonic CNS in *Drosophila* (A-C) and vertebrates (D-F). (A) Segmental topography of the *Drosophila* embryo at the phylotypic stage of development (stage 11). The scheme represents a flat preparation (anterior to the top), in which the head capsule has been opened dorsally. The pregnathal (from anterior to posterior: labral [Lr], ocular [Oc], antennal [Anl], intercalary [Ic]) and gnathal (mandibular [Md], maxillary [Mx], labial [La]) head segments are indicated on the right side. On the left side, the primordium of the CNS is highlighted in light grey (P, protocerebrum; D, deutocerebrum; T, tritocerebrum; Vnc, ventral nerve cord). B) The *Drosophila* embryonic brain develops from the procephalic neurogenic region of the ectoderm, which gives rise to a bilaterally symmetrical array of about 105 neural stem cells (neuroblasts). Shown is the left half of a head flat preparation (framed in A) including the complete brain neuroblast pattern. The colour code distinguishes between the neuroblast of the protocerebrum, (P, light brown), deutocerebrum (D, median brown) and tritocerebrum (T, dark brown); neuroblasts of the mandibular segment are also indicated (Md, grey). C) Morphology of the CNS in the late embryo (stage 17; lateral view, anterior to the left). D) Anterior part of the vertebrate CNS at the neural plate stage (anterior to the top). Indicated are the presumptive areas of the forebrain including the telencepahlon (Te) and diencephalon (Di), caudally followed by the midbrain (mesencephalon, Me), hindbrain (rhombencephalon, Rh), and the spinal cord (Sp). The notochord (N, dark grey) underlies the midline of the neural plate. Prechordal plate (Pcp) mesoderm underlies the embryonic ventral forebrain. E) Morphology of the vertebrate brain at about embryonic day 10 (mouse; lateral view, anterior to the left). F) As schematically shown in the coronal cross section (framed in E), the telencephalon can be subdivided from ventral to dorsal into three domains: the medial ganglionic eminence (Mge), the lateral ganglionic eminence (Lge) and the Cortex (Ctx). Further abbreviations: CL, clypeolabrum; Fg, foregut; Oa, optic lobe anlagen.

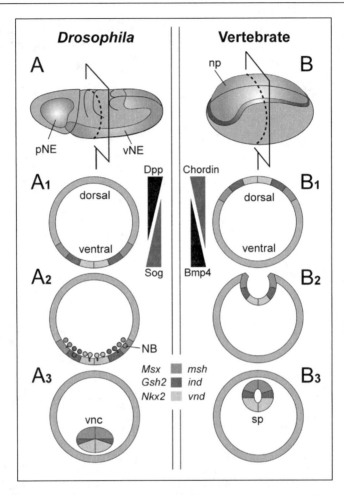

Figure 2. Expression of Dpp/ BMP4 and Sog/Chordin as well as of the columnar genes support the inversion of the DV body axis. Simplified schemes of cross sections through the trunk of developing *Drosophila* and vertebrate embryos (indicated by frames in A,B; neurogenic ectoderm highlighted in brown) during successive stages of development (A1-A3 and B1-B3, respectively). A1, B1) The border between nonneurogenic (grey) and neurogenic ectoderm (coloured) becomes defined by gradients of the antagonistically acting factors Short gastrulation (Sog)/Chordin (both in blue) and Decapentaplegic (Dpp)/Bone morphogenetic protein 4 (Bmp4) (both in red). The ectodermal region expressing *sog/chordin* forms the neuroectoderm, which is dorsal in vertebrates but ventral in *Drosophila*. DV patterning within the *Drosophila* neuroectoderm is achieved by the activity of the columnar genes: *msh*, *ind* and *vnd* (as indicated by the colour code), expressed in longitudinal columns at lateral, intermediate and ventral sites, respectively. A set of homologous genes *Msx*, *Gsh2* and *Nkx2*, is expressed in the vertebrate neuroectoderm in a corresponding medio-lateral sequence. A2, B2) Two different modes of morphogenesis are apparent during ongoing development: The *Drosophila* neuroectoderm gives rise to neuroblasts (NB), which delaminate towards the interior of the embryo to form the ventral nerve cord (vnc). The vertebrate neuroectoderm invaginates to form the dorsal neural tube. A3, B3) In the vertebrate spinal cord (sp) the columnar genes are nevertheless expressed in the same dorsoventral order as in the *Drosophila* ventral nerve cord. Further abbreviations: np, neural plate; vNE, ventral neuroectoderm; pNE, procephalic neuroectoderm.

protein 4 (BMP4), respectively, basically serve the same function.[4] In both species, the region in which *sog/Chordin* is expressed forms the neuroectoderm. Since the neuroectoderm is ventral in arthropods but dorsal in vertebrates, this has supported the hypothesis that the dorsoventral (DV) body axis became inverted during chordate evolution. This concept suggests a monophyletic origin and thus, homology of the CNS in protostomes and deuterostomes.[4-6]

Remarkably, despite the clear structural differences in the mature CNS, corresponding DV subdomains within arthropod and vertebrate neuroectoderm express homologous genes (known as "columnar" genes; described below). This suggests that aspects of DV patterning of the neuroectoderm have been evolutionarily conserved as well, which further supports homology of the arthropod and vertebrate CNS.

The less complex truncal nervous systems in *Drosophila* and vertebrates (mouse, chick, frog) have provided useful models to study the mechanisms of patterning and the generation of neural cell diversity. Many of the developmental processes that underlie NB formation, cell fate specification and pattern formation have been extensively studied in this more accessible part of the CNS (for a review see refs. 7-11). How cell diversity and patterning are achieved in the brain of both animal phyla is less well understood.

Here, we compare recent findings on mechanisms that specify DV fates in the early (embryonic) brain of *Drosophila* and vertebrates and compare these mechanisms with those acting in the truncal CNS.

DV Patterning of the Truncal Part of the CNS in *Drosophila* and Vertebrates

DV Patterning of the VNC in Drosophila

In *Drosophila*, the truncal neuroectoderm gives rise to the clearly metamerically organized VNC, which comprises 8 abdominal, 3 thoracic and 3 gnathal segmental units (neuromeres). The primordium of the VNC (neuroectoderm and NBs) is subdivided along the DV axis into adjacent longitudinal columns mainly by the activity of three homeobox genes (columnar genes). *ventral nervous system defective (vnd)* is expressed in the ventral, *intermediate neuroblasts defective (ind)* in the intermediate and *muscle segment homeobox (msh; Drop [Dr]*—FlyBase) in the dorsal neuroectodermal column (Fig. 3A).[12-18] Onset of their expression is at the blastoderm stage.

The genetic mechanisms establishing and maintaining the sharp borders between the domains of columnar gene expression in the VNC have been explored in detail. The columnar genes interact in a hierarchical cascade of transcriptional repression (also known as "ventral dominance"[19]) according to which *vnd* represses *ind* (and *msh*) in the ventral column and *ind* represses *msh* in the intermediate column. Thus, Vnd determines the ventral border of the Ind domain and Ind the ventral border of the Msh domain. The ventral border of the Vnd domain is defined by the mesoderm-specific genes *twist* and *snail* (for a review see refs. 20, 21). It is less clear how their dorsal borders are established. *msh* expression seems to be dorsally confined by the repressive activity of graded levels of Dpp and *vnd* expression by the Dorsal gradient, which activates *vnd*.[22] The dorsal border of *ind* expression may be formed by the limited activity of *Epidermal growth factor receptor (Egfr)* and Dorsal,[21] but also by the activity of spatially localized repressors, which are yet unknown.[23] Egfr activity in the ventral and intermediate column regulates the fate of NBs derived from these columns and is further necessary for the maintenance of *vnd* expression in the ventral column.[24-26] Furthermore, positional information provided by Dpp/BMP signalling contributes to patterning the neuroectoderm by repressing columnar genes in a threshold-dependent fashion.[27]

Columnar genes encode key regulators of NB identity and each column thereby gives rise to a population of distinctly specified NBs. However, whereas *vnd, ind* and *Egfr* have also been shown to be crucial for the formation of NBs in their respective column, this role appears dispensable for *msh* (for a review see ref. 20).

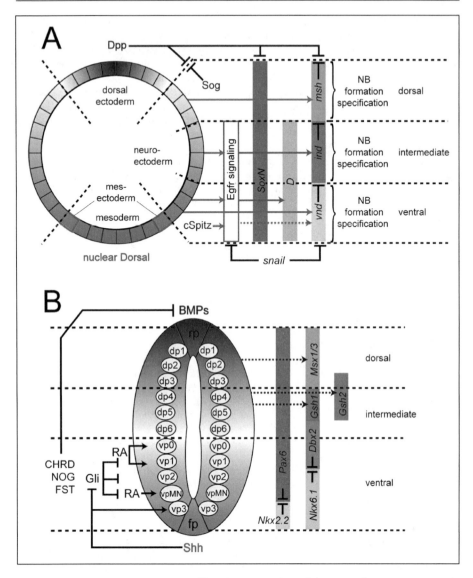

Figure 3. Genetic interactions controlling DV patterning of the truncal nervous system in
Drosophila and vertebrates. A) Schematic cross section through a *Drosophila* embryo at the
blastodermal stage. Intensity of red colour indicates gradient of Decapentaplegic (Dpp) which
in the dorsal ectoderm decreases from dorsal to ventral. Dpp is ventrally confined by repressive
activity of Short gastrulation (Sog). Intensity of blue colour indicates the gradient of nuclear
Dorsal protein, which increases from dorsal to ventral. Within the neuroectoderm, the proper
spatial domains of columnar gene expression are regulated by transcriptional repression: *vnd*
represses *ind* (and *msh*) in the ventral and *ind* represses *msh* in the intermediate neuroectoderm. Vnd and Epidermal growth factor receptor (Egfr) are ventrally delimited by repressive
activity of *snail* (from the mesoderm). Msh and SoxNeuro (SoxN) are dorsally repressed by
Dpp. Cleaved Spitz (cSpitz) emanating from mesectodermal cells (framed in pink) activates
EGFR signalling. Nuclear Dorsal activates *vnd*, *Egfr* and *msh* in a concentration-dependent
manner. Figure legend continued on following page.

Figure 3, continued from previous page. Egfr signaling in turn activates *ind* and *dichaete* (*D*) and is necessary for maintainence of *vnd*. Factors expressed in the ventral, intermediate and dorsal columns are necessary for proper formation and specification of neuroblasts (NB) in the respective domains (however, *msh* is dispensable for formation of dorsal NBs). B) Schematic cross section through an early neural tube, in which dorsal (dp1-6) and ventral neural progenitor domains (vp0-3, vpMN) developing within the ventricular zone are distinguished and some main genetic interactions which lead to their proper specification are indicated. These progenitor domains express distinct combinations of transcription factors and generate interneurons (dp1-6, vp0-3) or motoneurons (vpMN). The concentration of Bone morphogenetic proteins (BMPs, intensity of red colour), secreted from the roof plate (rp) decreases from dorsal to ventral. Patterning of dorsal and intermediate-type neural progenitors requires inductive activity of BMPs. Conversely, the gradient of Sonic hedgehog (Shh, intensity of grey colour), secreted from the floor plate (fp), decreases from ventral to dorsal. The Shh gradient is interpreted to establish the domains of ventral neuroblasts (vp0-3, vpMN). Shh also prevents the formation of the repressor form of GLI-Krüppel family member 3 (Gli), which inhibits specification of ventral progenitors domains (vp1, vp2, vpMN). Retinoid acid (RA) is involved in specification of the ventral neuroblast domains (vp0, vp1, vpMN) as well. Specification of ventral fates involves additionally the activity of BMP antagonists (Chordin [CHRD], Noggin [NOG], Follistatin [FST]). The ventral progenitor domains are confined by selective cross-repression of homeodomain proteins (as shown on the right): *Nkx2.2* and *Nkx6.1* complementarily cross-repress *Paired box 6* (*Pax6*) and *Developing brain homeobox 2* (*Dbx2*), respectively. Domains of neuroblasts in the dorsal half of the neural tube are specified by the activity of *Msx1/3* (expressed in dorsal dp1-3), *Gsh1/2* (expressed in intermediate-like dp3-5) and by the cross-repressive activity of basic helix-loop-helix proteins (such as Math1, Ngn1, Mash1, which are not indicated in the scheme). *Msx* genes and *Gsh2* act downstream of BMP signalling. Note the partial overlap of *Gsh2* and dorsal *Msx1/3* expression suggesting that *Gsh2* does not repress *Msx* genes, which contrasts the situation in *Drosophila*.

A Comparison with DV Patterning of the Spinal Cord in Vertebrates

Vertebrate genes closely related to *vnd* (*Nkx2.1, Nkx2.2*), *ind* (*Gsh1, Gsh2*) and *msh* (*Msx1, Msx2, Msx3*) are engaged in DV patterning of the developing neural plate (Fig. 2) (for a review see refs. 3, 21). However, compared to *Drosophila*, the genetic interactions which establish their domains of expression are less clear since the analysis in vertebrates is hampered by the large number of extrinsic signalling molecules involved and the inherent complexity of the genetic network due to the existence of multiple family members. For example, the *Msx* gene family in mouse comprises three copies of an ancestral *msh/Msx* gene.[28-30]

Although the spatial expression of the columnar genes in the neural tube closely mirrors the situation in *Drosophila*, there are apparent differences regarding the signalling mechanisms that act upstream. The floorplate/notochord at ventral and the roofplate at dorsal midline position of the developing neural tube represent two signalling centres, which induce (noncell-autonomously) dorsal and ventral neural fates. Similar to the floorplate, the mesectodermal ventral midline in *Drosophila* (which is specified by *single minded* and *Egfr*) operates as a signalling centre and plays an important role in the determination of cell fate in the lateral CNS and later in axon pathfinding.[31-33] However, in vertebrates, the signalling molecule secreted by the floor plate is Sonic hedgehog (Shh), a member of the hedgehog (*hh*) gene family. Graded Shh activates (or represses) the expression of various interacting homeobox genes (among which are the *vnd* homologs *Nkx2.1* and *Nkx2.2*, as well as *Nkx6.1*) and specifies the fates of neural progenitors in the ventral neural tube (vp0-3, vpMN; Fig. 3B)[34] (for a review see refs. 8,35). This contrasts the situation in *Drosophila*, in which the VNC is patterned (1) by *Dorsal* and *Egfr*, which induce *vnd* and *ind* (see above)[22] and (2) by the TGFα homologue Spitz, which is secreted by the ventral midline and leads to graded activation of Egfr in the neuroectoderm.[36,37] *Hh*, on the other hand, is expressed in segmental stripes orthogonal to the midline and controls cell fate within the ventral midline[38], but does not induce ventral-specific patterning genes in the adjacent neuroectoderm.

Much less is known about patterning and specification of dorsal and intermediate neuroblasts which descend from the dorsal half of the neural tube. In mouse, all three members of the *Msx* gene family are expressed in dorsalmost neuroblasts. While patterns of *Msx1* and *Msx2* expression are largely overlapping in several nonneural tissues as well, *Msx3* is exclusively restricted to the dorsal column of neural progenitors[39] (for a review see ref. 30). *Msx* expression in the dorsal column is determined by molecules of the TGF-β family secreted from the roof plate, among which are the Dpp-related BMP2/4. BMP2/4 activate and seem to define both the dorsal and ventral border of *Msx* expression.[40] This appeared to be in contrast to *Drosophila*, where Dpp represses *msh* and thus defines only the dorsal border of its expression.[22] However, it has recently been reported that graded Dpp activity helps establish the *msh/ind* and the *ind/vnd* borders as well by repressing *msh*, *ind* and *vnd* in a threshold-dependent fashion and that BMPs act in a similar fashion in chick neural plate explants.[27] *Gsh1* and *Gsh2* are expressed in an intermediate column in the neural tube. Both genes are necessary for fate specification of intermediate progenitors (in the progenitor domains dp3-5; Fig. 3B). *Gsh2* is proposed to act downstream of BMP/TGFß signalling.[41] In *Drosophila* normal level of *ind* expression critically depends on *Egfr* signalling. Although an *Egfr* homolog has been identified in zebrafish, it does not seem to have an instructive function in neural patterning of the spinal cord[42] (for a review see ref. 21). A further difference is that the expression domain of *Gsh2* partly overlaps with that of the *Msx* genes and that expression of *Msx1* and *Msx3* is unchanged in *Gsh2* single or *Gsh1/2* double mutants. This indicates that *Gsh2* cannot repress *Msx1/3*, opposite to the *Drosophila* VNC, where *ind* clearly represses *msh*. On the other hand, in both the vertebrate spinal cord and the *Drosophila* VNC, *Msx/msh* does not repress *Gsh/ind*.[18,41]

Interestingly, it has been shown that mouse *Gsh1* (and *Nkx2.2*) does not function in *Drosophila* VNC development, suggesting that functional domains have become distinct over time. In contrast, function of zebrafish *Nkx6.1* and fly *Nkx6* seems conserved since in both species overexpression of the respective ortholog leads to the induction of supernumerary motoneurons.[43]

Further factors involved in the specification of intermediate identities remain to be resolved, as for example signals involved in fate specification of "dp6" progenitors. Such signals may include retinoid acid, which is also necessary for proper development of the adjacent ventral neural progenitors (for a review see ref. 44). In the vertebrate neural tube, gaps have been observed between the expression domains of the columnar genes, raising the possibility that other genes might fill in these gaps.[18] It has been suggested that, in addition to the columns of *msh/Msx*, *ind/Gsh* and *vnd/Nkx2*, the early neural tube includes at least a fourth DV column which expresses the *developing brain homeobox2* (*Dbx2*) gene.[41,45,46] The *Dbx2* expression domain is positioned between the intermediate *Gsh1/Gsh2* and ventral *Nkx6.1* column and includes the "dp6" progenitors. Its ventral border is determined by repressive activity of *Nkx6.1*, but the factor controlling its dorsal border is unknown. However, the *Drosophila Dbx* homolog, *H2.0*, although expressed in subsets of NBs and progeny cells, does not seem to be involved in DV specification of NBs since it is not expressed in the truncal neuroectoderm.[41]

DV Patterning of the Brain in *Drosophila*

The *Drosophila* larval brain develops from the procephalic neuroectoderm (pNE) which gives rise to a bilaterally symmetrical array of about 100 embryonic NBs.[47] Presumably all embryonic NBs become postembryonically reactivated to form the adult brain,[48] whereas in the VNC postembryonic mitotic activity becomes restricted to segment-specific subpopulations of NBs. The pattern of embryonic brain NBs neither exhibits an ordered segmental assembly, nor morphologically distinct subdivisions into anteroposterior rows or dorsoventral columns, as is at least transiently the case in the VNC. Accordingly, the segmental composition of the brain is not obvious. The brain is subdivided, from posterior to anterior, into the tritocerebrum, deutocerebrum and protocerebrum (Fig. 1A-C). The embryonic trito- and deutocerebrum correspond to one neuromere each, deriving form the intercalary and antennal segment, respectively. There is evidence that the protocerebrum may consist of two neuromeres, a large one deriving from the ocular segment and a small remnant of the labral segment.[49,50] Likewise, DV regionalisation of the early embryonic brain is not overt and the underlying patterning mechanisms are only rudimentarily understood. The columnar genes are expressed in distinct areas of the pNE and the developing brain. Although their expression is consistent with their role in DV patterning being principally conserved in the procephalon, there are also significant differences in their patterns of expression as compared to the trunk.

Expression of Columnar Genes in the Early Embryonic Brain

At the gastrula stage, *vnd* is expressed in the ventral pNE, covering the prospective ventral parts of the trito-, deuto- and protocerebrum. While Vnd in the trunk, is maintained within a continuous ventral neuroectodermal column during subsequent stages, *vnd* expression in the early brain is highly dynamic. It becomes progressively confined to three separate ventral domains at the posterior border of the trito-, deuto- and protocerebrum, encompassing different numbers of NBs and progeny cells (Fig. 4A).[51,52] *msh* is expressed in the dorsal neuroectoderm of the intercalary and antennal segments which give rise to trito- and deutocerebral NBs. It is not expressed in the primordium of the protocerebrum. In the trunk, *ind* is expressed in a continuous column of intermediate neuroectoderm, whereas in the procephalic neuroectoderm it is found in three separate spots (in the intercalary, antennal and ocular segment). The intercalary and antennal *ind* spot are located at intermediate position between the dorsal Msh and ventral Vnd domain. Opposed to that, the ocular *ind* spot is spatially clearly separated from the ventral Vnd domain (and *msh* is not expressed). Due to the insulated expression of *ind*, the intercalary and antennal domains of *msh* and *vnd* expression share a common border at sites lacking an intervening *ind* domain.[50]

Another conspicuous difference to the trunk (and to the TC and DC as well) is that a large amount of the protocerebral NBs (more than 50%) does not express any of the three columnar genes (Fig. 4A).[50] Similarly, in the vertebrate spinal cord gaps have been detected between the domains of columnar gene expression.[18] Thus, DV patterning of the protocerebral primordia of the brain anlagen requires factors additional to those encoded by the columnar genes. Candidate genes might include *Egfr*,[24-26] the Sox genes *SoxNeuro* and *Dicheate*,[53-55] the *Nkx2.1* homologous gene *scarecrow*,[56] the *Nkx6* family related gene *Nk6*,[43,57] or perhaps the *Dbx* homologous gene, *H2.0*.[58] Most of these, except *scarecrow* and *H2.0*, are known to have a function in fate specification and/or formation of NBs in the trunk. *Egfr*, both *Sox* genes and *Nk6* are expressed in the pNE before and during the phase of NB formation[43,57] (J. Seibert and R. Urbach, unpublished observations), however, their role in the formation/specification of brain NBs is yet unknown.

Segment-Specific Regulation of Columnar Genes

Recent reports gave first insights into the interactions and function of columnar genes during DV patterning of the embryonic brain.[51,52] Although principally the same DV patterning genes operate in large parts of the pNE, their regulation reveals segment-specific differences both among the brain segments and compared to the trunk (Fig. 4B).

For example, contrary to the trunk, in *vnd* mutant background derepression of *ind* within the ventral pNE does not occur in the antennal segment. Instead, *ind* expression is completely absent, indicating that, at least in this part of the pNE and brain, *vnd* is necessary for activation and/or maintenance of *ind* rather than for its repression (as in the trunk). This is supported by the finding that ectopic expression of *vnd* does not repress *ind* in the antennal segment. The ocular *ind* spot is often ventrally expanded in the absence of Vnd, which is reminiscent of the situation in the trunk. However, in the wildtype, the ocular *ind* spot does not adjoin the ventral domain of *vnd* expression. Hence, a ventral expansion of ocular *ind* in *vnd* mutants cannot be due to the lack of repression by Vnd and may be regulated noncell-autonomously.[52]

Moreover, in the absence of Vnd, expression of *msh* reveals segment-specific differences. Its expression is ectopically expanded into the ventral pNE of the intercalary and antennal segment, due to lack of repression by Vnd and Ind. This is not the case in the neuroectoderm of the protocerebrum and trunk. In the latter *ind* is derepressed instead of *msh*.

Taken together, expression and interactions of columnar genes (i.e., the cascade of transcriptional repression which establishes the ventral border of the *msh* and *ind* domain) appears to be conserved in the most posterior brain, the tritocerebrum. Although the expression of columnar genes is to some extent conserved in the deutocerebrum as well, their genetic interactions are more derived in the deuto- and protocerebrum.[52] So far it is not settled how these segment-specific differences

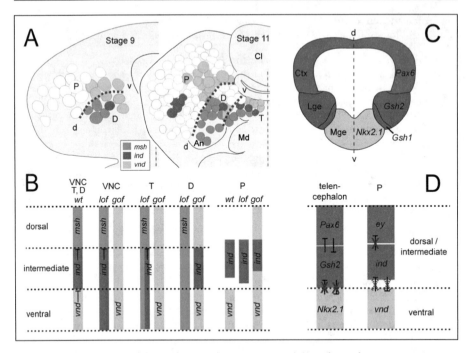

Figure 4. DV patterning of the embryonic brain in *Drosophila* and vertebrates. A) Expression of the columnar genes *msh*, *ind* and *vnd* (see colour code) in neuroblasts of the tritocerebrum (T), deutocerebrum (D) and protocerebrum (P) at the embryonic stages 9 and 11. Each scheme represents the left half of a head flat preparation (compare with Fig. 1B) including the full complement of neuroblasts at the respective stages (encircled). Red stippled lines indicate borders between neuromeres. *vnd* is expressed in ventral (v), *ind* in intermediate and *msh* in dorsal (d) neuroblasts. Vnd becomes progressively expressed at the posterio-ventral border of the trito-, deuto- and protocerebrum. Msh expression is confined to dorsal neuroblasts of the trito- and deutocerebrum, but is not found in the protocerebrum. Expression of *ind* is confined to three separate spots of neuroblasts in the trito-, deuto- and protocerebrum. Note that domains of Msh and Vnd share common borders at sites where expression of *ind* is lacking. Further abbreviations: An, antennal; CL, clypeolabral; Md; madibular appendage. B) Diagramm summarizing the segment-specific differences in the regulatory interactions of columnar genes in the ventral nerve cord (VNC), trito- (T), deuto- (D) and protocerebrum (P) in wildtype (*wt*), *vnd* loss-of-function (*lof*) and *vnd* gain-of-function (*gof*) embryos (for details see text). C) Schematic of a coronal section of the mouse telencephalon at about embryonic day 10 (compare with Fig. 1F). The *vnd* homolog *Nkx2.1* is expressed in the most ventral area, the medial ganglionic eminence (Mge), the *ind* homolog *Gsh2* in the lateral ganglionic eminence (Lge) and the *eyeless* (*ey*) homolog *Pax6* in the dorsal cortex (Ctx), where, similar to the situation in *Drosophila*, Msx genes are not expressed. D) Diagramm comparing the regulatory interactions between *Pax6*, *Gsh2* and *Nkx2.1* in the vertebrate telencephalon with those of the homologous genes *ey*, *ind* and *vnd* in the *Drosophila* protocerebrum (P). For details see text. In the vertebrate telencephalon, opposite to the situation in the spinal cord, *Pax6* and *Gsh2* mutually repress one another (compare with Fig. 3B). *Gsh2* and *Nkx2.1* do not act in a cross-repressive manner (as indicated by red crossed repression symbols).[65] Similarly, *vnd* and *ind* in the protocerebrum do not directly interfere (indicated by stippled red crossed repression symbols). Although the altered extent of the *ind* expression domain in *vnd lof* and *gof* backgrounds indicates regulatory interactions (see Fig. 4B), they must be noncell-autonomous, since the normal *vnd* and *ind* expression domains do not abut each other. Expression of *ey* (and *twin of eyeless*, not indicated) is unaffected in *ind* mutants, suggesting that, in contrast to the situation in the telencephalon, *ind* does not repress *ey* (indicated by red crossed repression symbol). It is not yet clear, if conversely, *ind* expression is affected in the absence of *ey* and/or *twin of eyeless*.

are regulated. It also remains to be clarified in how far other factors (e.g., those described above) genetically interfere with the columnar genes in the pNE and may establish the gene-specific extent of their expression both in the DV and AP axis.

Role of Columnar Genes in Formation of Brain NBs

In *vnd* mutants, ventral brain NBs are largely absent indicating that, similar to the situation in the trunk, *vnd* promotes formation of NBs. In the absence of Vnd, cell death is increased and acts at the level of both, neuroectodermal progenitors cells and NBs.[52] It is not yet resolved if the reduction in ventral NBs is solely due to an increase in cell death or involves other factors known to be engaged in NB formation, such as proneural genes of the *AS*-complex (*acheate, scute, lethal of scute* [*l'sc*]; for a review see ref. 59). In the trunk, there is evidence that *vnd* interacts with proneural genes, but may also have additional function in promoting NB formation. Accordingly, in *vnd* mutant embryos, *l'sc* is still expressed in ventral proneural clusters, although the respective NBs will not form (e.g., NB5-2).[13,60] In the pNE, genes of the *AS*-complex are expressed in large proneural domains and the *acheate* and *l'sc* domain seem to overlap with the domain of *vnd* expression, compatible with a genetic interaction.[47,61] However, in *vnd* mutant embryos no substantial difference to the wildtype expression pattern of *l'sc* transcript is observed (R.U., unpublished observation), suggesting that, if *vnd* has proneural activity, it is rather independent of *l'sc*. Nevertheless, the expression of another proneural gene, *atonal* (in the pNE normally expressed in proneural clusters and developing sensory precursors of the hypopharyngeal-/latero-hypopharyngeal organ), is often missing indicating its dependence on Vnd.[52] Thus far it is unclear if *msh, ind* and *Egfr* exert a similar function in brain NB formation. Whereas *Egfr* mutant embryos exhibit strong defects in the number and pattern of brain NBs, they appear rather unaffected in *msh* mutants (J.Seibert and R.U., unpublished observation), indicating that at least *msh* does not play a role in brain NB formation. *Egfr* signalling has also been shown to be necessary for the proper development of medial brain structures deriving from the head midline, which behaves like the mesectoderm in the trunk.[62] Placode-like groups of cells from the head midline invaginate and contribute subpopulations of cells to the brain.[61] Loss of *Egfr* signalling results in severe reduction or absence of the respective head midline derivatives.

Role of vnd in Specification of Brain NBs

In the trunk, evidence has been provided, that the set of genes expressed within a proneural cluster specifies the individual identity of the NB it gives rise to. Such a combinatorial code, which is unique for each NB, is provided mainly by the superimposition of the acitivity of DV patterning genes and segment polarity genes (AP axis) and a number of other factors (for a review see refs. 9, 20, 63). Most of these genes are also expressed in specific procephalic neuroectodermal domains before NBs delaminate, implying that these genes might be required for specification of individual brain NBs as well.[64] Analysis of an array of such NB identity genes in *vnd* loss- and gain-of function backgrounds indicates that, similar to the situation in the trunk, *vnd* influences their expression already in the pNE, before the formation of NBs.[52]

In *vnd* loss-of-function background, dorsal-specific gene expression is derepressed in the ventral pNE and descending NBs and conversely, ventral-specific gene expression is lost, suggesting a ventral-to-dorsal transformation of the mutant ventral pNE and residual ventral NBs. This indicates that *vnd* normally activates genes specific for the ventral pNE and represses genes specific for dorsal pNE and is required for fate specification of ventral brain NBs. This is further supported by the production of ectopic glial cells derived from transfated ventral NBs in the trito- and deutocerebrum, which normally is a specific trait of dorsal brain NBs. Later in embryogenesis a severe loss of neural tissue associated with increased apoptotic activity has been observed in the tritocerebrum, presumably as a consequence of identity changes imposed on *vnd* deficient NB lineages.[51]

Upon *vnd* overexpression, there is a wide-ranging loss of dorsal-specific gene activity in the dorsal pNE and NBs, but a largely unaffected ventral-specific gene activity in ventral parts. Moreover, there is evidence for a partial dorsal-to-ventral transformation of dorsal parts of the pNE and corresponding NBs, which indicates that Vnd is not only necessary but to some extent also sufficient to induce ventral traits.

A Comparison with DV Regionalization of the Vertebrate Telencephalon

The telencephalon derives from paired evaginations of the anterior forebrain that constitute the most complex structures of the vertebrate CNS. Progress has been made in understanding the early regional patterning of the telencephalon, although the present knowledge about its DV regionalization is still rudimentary. The telencephalon can be subdivided into a dorsal or pallial and a ventral or subpallial territory and the subpallium further into the lateral ganglionic eminence (LGE) and a ventralmost part, the medial ganglionic eminence (MGE) (Fig. 1). The pallium gives rise to the cortex, the subpallium to the basal ganglia. The future telencephalic territories can be defined early in development by the expression of *Nkx2.1* in the ventral MGE and *Gsh1, Gsh2* in the intermediate LGE, resembling the expression of *vnd* and *ind* in the anlagen of the *Drosophila* brain. *Pax6*, the homolog of *Drosophila eyeless* (*ey*), is expressed in the dorsal telencephalon (Fig. 4C). *Pax6* is involved in the specification of pallial identity (for a review see refs. 66, 67) instead of *Msx* genes which are not expressed in the telencephalon. Interestingly, *Drosophila ey* is likewise preferentially expressed in dorsal/intermediate NBs of the protocerebrum, which lack *msh* expression[64], suggesting that *ey* may to some extent play the role of *msh* in the anterior brain. In the telencephalon, *Nkx2.1, Gsh2* and *Pax6* are complementary expressed, provide some of the earliest markers for the respective territories and are key regulators for their normal development (for a review see ref. 67).

Genetic Interactions of Columnar Genes

Although a conserved set of homeobox genes is expressed at corresponding DV positions in the brains of arthropods and vertebrates, there are differences in their genetic interactions. In the telencephalon *Gsh2* and *Pax6* cross-repress each other, which results in the formation of a sharp border between the dorsal and intermediate domains (Fig. 4C, D). Accordingly, in *Pax6* mutant mice there is evidence for a dorsal-to-ventral transformation of dorsal (pallial) structures, which is opposite to the phenotype in *Gsh2* mutants.[68-70] This behaviour is specific to the telencephalon and not observed in the spinal cord. Similarly, in the *Drosophila* protocerebrum and deutocerebrum, *ey* and *ind* are largely expressed in complementary subsets of NBs.[64] However, *ey* expression does not seem to depend on Ind, since it does not expand ventrally in *ind* mutants (R.U., unpublished observations), as opposed to *Pax6* in the telencephalon of *Gsh2* mutants.[69] In the tritocerebrum, opposite to the anterior brain, *ey* is coexpressed with *ind*[64], resembling the situation in the vertebrate spinal cord, in which the domains of *Pax6* and *Gsh2* overlap.[41,67] It is worth noting, that *Drosophila* has a second *Pax6* gene, *twin of eyeless* (*toy*), which is largely expressed in the protocerebrum. However, since *ind* is coexpressed with *toy* in the protocerebrum[64], it is unlikely that *ind* and *toy* (instead of *ey*) genetically behave in a way similar to *Pax6* and *Gsh2* in the telencephalon.

Among the columnar genes, particularly the family of *Nkx/vnd* genes seems to be well conserved in terms of expression and function. In mice carrying a deletion of *Nkx2.1*, a substantial loss of ventral, especially of forebrain structures has been observed. The residual ventral (subpallial) structures become transfated into dorsal striatal structures.[71] An interesting correlation between the regulation of columnar genes in the vertebrate telencephalon and *Drosophila* deuto- and protocerebrum is that *Nkx2.1* and *vnd* do not repress the expression of *Gsh* and *ind*, respectively. Accordingly, in *Nkx2.1* knockout mouse, as well as in *Drosophila vnd* mutants, the expression of *Gsh2/ind* in these brain regions is not ventrally expanded[51,71], contrary to findings made in the truncal CNS (for a review see ref. 21). Instead of intermediate *Gsh/ind*, dorsal-specific marker genes are derepressed in ventralmost areas of the early brain; among these are *Pax6*, in the vertebrate telencephalon and *ey* (to a minor extent) and especially *msh* in the *Drosophila* deuto-and tritocerebrum. Together, this suggests that in *Nkx2.1/vnd* mutant background, residual ventral brain territories undergo a ventral-to-dorsal rather than a ventral-to-intermediate transformation, the latter being observed in the truncal CNS of both species.[13,73,74]

Genetic Factors Upstream of the Columnar Genes

Several extrinsic signalling molecules are involved in DV patterning of the telencephalon, among which are BMPs, Wnts, Gli, FGFs, Nodal, retinoic acid and the central player Shh (for a review see refs. 44, 67, 75). The mechanisms by which Shh induces DV fate might differ between spinal cord and brain. Whereas in the spinal cord, the fates induced by Shh are concentration-dependent, Shh-induced fates in the telencephalon depend on timing rather than concentration (for a review see ref. 67). In the telencephalon, the source of secreted Shh is (among others) the prechordal plate, a mesodermal derivative. Remarkably, the *Drosophila* homolog, Hh, secreted from the head mesoderm and foregut, acts on brain morphogenesis by regulating size and apoptosis. *hh*, expressed in the foregut, appears to mediate these effects via the Hh receptor *patched* (expressed in brain cells surrounding the foregut). These similarities may indicate an ancient mechanism of brain patterning via induction.[76] In how far other extrinsic signalling molecules are involved in DV patterning of the *Drosophila* brain remains to be shown.

Conclusions

A conserved set of columnar genes (*msh/Msx, ind/Gsh, vnd/Nkx*) is involved in DV regionalization of the brain and truncal CNS in vertebrates and arthropods (*Drosophila*). The expression of columnar genes in the brain differs from the truncal CNS in both animal phyla. Remarkably, the brain-specific expression of columnar genes exibits striking parallels between *Drosophila* and mouse in that the anterior borders of their domains are corresponding: Expression of *vnd/Nkx2* extends most rostrally, followed by *ind/Gsh1* and finally by *msh/Msx3* (for a review see ref. 77). Thus, the expression of columnar genes in the brain is, to some extent, evolutionarily conserved, not only along the DV axis but also along the AP axis.

Moreover, brain-specific interactions among columnar genes bear some similarities between vertebrates and *Drosophila*. For example, *Gsh/ind* are not repressed by *Nkx2.1/vnd* and expression of dorsal factors, instead of intermediate, is expanded into ventral domains in *vnd/Nkx2* mutant brains. This suggests that at least part of the genetic mechanisms governing DV fate in the brain have been conserved as well. Differences may become more obvious at the level of upstream regulating factors. However, in vertebrates, as well as in *Drosophila*, the genetic basis underlying DV regionalization of the brain is far from being understood. The *Drosophila* brain, due to its comparatively small size, allowing resolution at the level of individually identified cells and to the powerful genetic and experimental tools available, provides a useful model system to study these mechanisms in detail. This will facilitate the clarification of the processes underlying DV regionalization in the brain of other organisms, including vertebrates.

Acknowledgements

We are grateful to Ana Rogulja-Ortmann for comments on the manuscript. This work was supported by the Deutsche Forschungsgemeinschaft and the EC.

References

1. Hartenstein V, Campos-Ortega JA. Early neurogenesis in wild-type Drosophila melanogaster. Roux's Archives of Developmental Biology 1984; 193:308-325.
2. Poulson DS. Histogenesis, organogenesis and differentiation in the embryo of Drosophila melanogaster Meigen. In: Demerec M, ed. Biology of Drosophila. New York: Wiley, 1950:168-274.
3. Arendt D, Nübler-Jung K. Comparison of early nerve cord development in insects and vertebrates. Development 1999; 126:2309-2325.
4. Holley SA, Jackson PD, Sasai Y et al. A conserved system for dorsal-ventral patterning in insects and vertebrates involving sog and chordin. Nature 1995; 376:249-253.
5. Arendt D, Nübler-Jung K. Dorsal or ventral: similarities in fate maps and gastrulation patterns in annelids, arthropods and chordates. Mech Dev 1997; 61:7-21.
6. De Robertis EM, Sasai Y. A common plan for dorsoventral patterning in Bilateria. Nature. 1996; 380:37-40.
7. Lumsden A, Krumlauf R. Patterning the vertebrate neuraxis. Science 1996; 274:1109-1115.
8. Jessell TM. Neuronal specification in the spinal cord: inductive signals and transcriptional codes. Nat Rev Genet 2000; 1:20-29.

9. Skeath JB, Thor S. Genetic control of Drosophila nerve cord development. Curr Opin Neurobiol 2003; 13:8-15.

10. Pearson BJ, Doe CQ. Specification of temporal identity in the developing nervous system. Annu Rev Cell Dev Biol 2004; 20:619-647.

11. Price SR, Briscoe J. The generation and diversification of spinal motor neurons: signals and responses. Mech Dev 2004; 121:1103-1115.

12. Buescher M, Chia W. Mutations in lottchen cause cell fate transformations in both neuroblast and glioblast lineages in the Drosophila embryonic central nervous system. Development 1997; 124:673-681.

13. Chu H, Parras C, White K et al. Formation and specification of ventral neuroblasts is controlled by vnd in Drosophila neurogenesis. Genes Dev 1998; 12:3613-3624.

14. D'Alessio M, Frasch M. msh may play a conserved role in dorsoventral patterning of the neuroectoderm and mesoderm. Mech Dev 1996; 58:217-231.

15. Isshiki T, Takeichi M, Nose A. The role of the msh homeobox gene during Drosophila neurogenesis: implication for the dorsoventral specification of the neuroectoderm. Development 1997; 124:3099-3109.

16. Jimenez F, Martin-Morris LE, Velasco L et al. vnd, a gene required for early neurogenesis of Drosophila, encodes a homeodomain protein. EMBO J 1995; 14:3487-3495.

17. Mellerick DM, Nirenberg M. Dorsal-ventral patterning genes restrict NK-2 homeobox gene expression to the ventral half of the central nervous system of Drosophila embryos. Dev Biol 1995; 171:306-316.

18. Weiss JB, Von Ohlen T, Mellerick DM et al. Dorsoventral patterning in the Drosophila central nervous system: the intermediate neuroblasts defective homeobox gene specifies intermediate column identity. Genes Dev 1998; 12:3591-3602.

19. Cowden J, Levine M. Ventral dominance governs sequential patterns of gene expression across the dorsal–ventral axis of the neuroectoderm in the Drosophila embryo. Dev Biol 2003; 262:335-349.

20. Skeath JB. At the nexus between pattern formation and cell-type specification: the generation of individual neuroblast fates in the Drosophila embryonic central nervous system. Bioessays 1999; 21:922-931.

21. Cornell RA, Ohlen TV. Vnd/nkx, ind/gsh and msh/msx: conserved regulators of dorsoventral neural patterning? Curr Opin Neurobiol 2000; 10:63-71.

22. von Ohlen T, Doe CQ. Convergence of dorsal, dpp and egfr signaling pathways subdivides the Drosophila neuroectoderm into three dorsal-ventral columns. Dev Biol 2000; 224:362-372.

23. Stathopoulos A, Levine M. Localized repressors delineate the neurogenic ectoderm in the early Drosophila embryo. Dev Biol 2005; 280:482-493.

24. Skeath JB. The Drosophila EGF receptor controls the formation and specification of neuroblasts along the dorsal-ventral axis of the Drosophila embryo. Development 1998; 125:3301-3312.

25. Yagi Y, Suzuki T, Hayashi S. Interaction between Drosophila EGF receptor and vnd determines three dorsoventral domains of the neuroectoderm. Development 1998; 125:3625-3633.

26. Udolph G, Urban J, Rüsing G et al. Differential effects of EGF receptor signalling on neuroblast lineages along the dorsoventral axis of the Drosophila CNS. Development 1998; 125:3292-3299.

27. Mizutani CM, Meyer N, Roelink H et al. Threshold-dependent BMP-mediated repression: A model for a conserved mechanism that pattern the neuroectoderm. PLOS Biology 2006; 4:e313.

28. Catron KM, Wang H, Hu G et al. Comparison of MSX-1 and MSX-2 suggests a molecular basis for functional redundancy. Mech Dev 1996; 55:185-199.

29. Wang W, Chen X, Xu H et al. Msx3: a novel murine homologue of the Drosophila msh homeobox gene restricted to the dorsal embryonic central nervous system. Mech Dev 1996; 58:203-215.

30. Ramos C, Robert B. msh/Msx gene family in neural development. Trends Genet 2005; 21:624-632.

31. Crews ST. Control of cell lineage-specific development and transcription by bHLH-PAS proteins. Genes Dev 1998; 12:607-620.

32. Kim IO, Kim IC, Kim S et al. CNS midline cells contribute to maintenance of the initial dorsoventral patterning of the Drosophila ventral neuroectoderm. J Neurobiol 2005; 62:397-405.

33. Jacobs JR. The midline glia of Drosophila: a molecular genetic model for the developmental functions of glia. Prog Neurobiol 2000; 62:475-508.

34. Ericson J, Muhr J, Placzek M et al. Sonic hedgehog induces the differentiation of ventral forebrain neurons: a common signal for ventral patterning within the neural tube. Cell 1995; 81:747-756.

35. Wilson L, Maden M. The mechanisms of dorsoventral patterning in the vertebrate neural tube. Dev Biol 2005; 282:1-13.

36. Golembo M, Raz E, Shilo BZ. The Drosophila embryonic midline is the site of Spitz processing and induces activation of the EGF receptor in the ventral ectoderm. Development 1996; 122:3363-3370.

37. Schweitzer R, Shilo BZ. A thousand and one roles for the Drosophila EGF receptor. Trends Genet 1997; 13:191-196.

38. Bossing T, Brand AH. Determination of cell fate along the anteroposterior axis of the Drosophila ventral midline. Development 2006; 133:1001-1012.

39. Liu Y, Helms AW, Johnson JE. Distinct activities of Msx1 and Msx3 in dorsal neural tube development. Development 2004; 131:1017-1028.
40. Suzuki A, Ueno N, Hemmati-Brivanlou A. Xenopus msx1 mediates epidermal induction and neural inhibition by BMP4. Development 1997; 124:3037-3044.
41. Kriks S, Lanuza GM, Mizuguchi R et al. Gsh2 is required for the repression of Ngn1 and specification of dorsal interneuron fate in the spinal cord. Development 2005; 132:2991-3002.
42. Strahle U, Jesuthasan S, Blader P et al. one-eyed pinhead is required for development of the ventral midline of the zebrafish (Danio rerio) neural tube. Genes Funct 1997; 1:131-148.
43. Cheesman SE, Layden MJ, Von Ohlen T et al. Zebrafish and fly Nkx6 proteins have similar CNS expression patterns and regulate motoneuron formation. Development 2004; 131:5221-5232.
44. Zhuang B, Sockanathan S. Dorsal-ventral patterning: a view from the top. Curr Opin Neurobiol 2006; 16:20-24.
45. Fjose A, Izpisua-Belmonte JC, Fromental-Ramain C et al. Expression of the zebrafish gene hlx-1 in the prechordal plate and during CNS development. Development 1994; 120:71-81.
46. Pierani A, Moran-Rivard L, Sunshine MJ et al. Control of interneuron fate in the developing spinal cord by the progenitor homeodomain protein Dbx1. Neuron 2001; 29:367-384.
47. Urbach R, Schnabel R, Technau GM. The pattern of neuroblast formation, mitotic domains and proneural gene expression during early brain development in Drosophila. Development 2003; 130:3589-3606.
48. Lee CY, Robinson KJ, Doe CQ. Lgl, Pins and aPKC regulate neuroblast self-renewal versus differentiation. Nature 2006; 439:594-598.
49. Schmidt-Ott U, Technau GM. Expression of en and wg in the embryonic head and brain of Drosophila indicates a refolded band of seven segment remnants. Development 1992; 116:111-125.
50. Urbach R, Technau GM. Segment polarity and D/V patterning gene expression reveals segmental organization of the Drosophila brain. Development 2003; 130:3607-3620.
51. Sprecher S, Urbach R, Technau GM et al. The columnar gene vnd is rquired for tritocerebral neuromere formation during embryonic brain development of Drosophila. Development 2006; 133:4331-4339.
52. Urbach R, Volland D, Seibert J et al. Segment-specific requirements for dorsoventral patterning genes during early brain development in Drosophila. Development 2006; 133:4315-4330.
53. Buescher M, Hing FS, Chia W. Formation of neuroblasts in the embryonic central nervous system of Drosophila melanogaster is controlled by SoxNeuro. Development 2002; 129:4193-4203.
54. Sanchez-Soriano N, Russell S. Regulatory mutations of the Drosophila Sox gene Dichaete reveal new functions in embryonic brain and hindgut development. Dev Biol 2000; 220:307-321.
55. Zhao G, Skeath JB. The Sox-domain containing gene Dichaete/fish-hook acts in concert with vnd and ind to regulate cell fate in the Drosophila neuroectoderm. Development 2002; 129:1165-1174.
56. Zaffran S, Das G, Frasch M. The NK-2 homeobox gene scarecrow (scro) is expressed in pharynx, ventral nerve cord and brain of Drosophila embryos. Mech Dev 2000; 94:237-241.
57. Uhler J, Garbern J, Yang L et al. Nk6, a novel Drosophila homeobox gene regulated by vnd. Mech Dev 2002; 116:105-116.
58. Barad M, Jack T, Chadwick R et al. A novel, tissue-specific, Drosophila homeobox gene. EMBO J 1988; 7:2151-2161.
59. Campos-Ortega JA. Genetic mechanisms of early neurogenesis in Drosophila melanogaster. Mol Neurobiol 1995; 10:75-89.
60. Skeath JB, Panganiban GF, Carroll SB. The ventral nervous system defective gene controls proneural gene expression at two distinct steps during neuroblast formation in Drosophila. Development 1994; 120:1517-1524.
61. Younossi-Hartenstein A, Nassif C, Green P et al. Early neurogenesis of the Drosophila brain. J Comp Neurol 1996; 370:313-329.
62. Dumstrei K, Nassif C, Abboud G et al. EGFR signaling is required for the differentiation and maintenance of neural progenitors along the dorsal midline of the Drosophila embryonic head. Development 1998; 125:3417-3426.
63. Bhat KM. Segment polarity genes in neuroblast formation and identity specification during Drosophila neurogenesis. Bioessays 1999; 21:472-485.
64. Urbach R, Technau GM. Molecular markers for identified neuroblasts in the developing brain of Drosophila. Development 2003; 130:3621-3637.
65. Wilson SW, Rubenstein JL. Induction and dorsoventral patterning of the telencephalon. Neuron 2000; 28:641-651.
66. Manuel M, Price DJ. Role of Pax6 in forebrain regionalization. Brain Res Bull 2005; 66:387-393.
67. Rallu M, Corbin JG, Fishell G. Parsing the prosencephalon. Nat Rev Neurosci 2002; 3:943-951.
68. Stoykova A, Treichel D, Hallonet M et al. Pax6 modulates the dorsoventral patterning of the mammalian telencephalon. J Neurosci 2000; 20:8042-8050.

69. Toresson H, Potter SS, Campbell K. Genetic control of dorsal-ventral identity in the telencephalon: opposing roles for Pax6 and Gsh2. Development 2000; 127:4361-4371.
70. Yun K, Potter S, Rubenstein JL. Gsh2 and Pax6 play complementary roles in dorsoventral patterning of the mammalian telencephalon. Development 2001; 128:193-205.
71. Sussel L, Marin O, Kimura S et al. Loss of Nkx2.1 homeobox gene function results in a ventral to dorsal molecular respecification within the basal telencephalon: evidence for a transformation of the pallidum into the striatum. Development 1999; 126:3359-3370.
72. Corbin JG, Rutlin M, Gaiano N et al. Combinatorial function of the homeodomain proteins Nkx2.1 and Gsh2 in ventral telencephalic patterning. Development 2003; 130:4895-4906.
73. Briscoe J, Sussel L, Serup P et al. Homeobox gene Nkx2.2 and specification of neuronal identity by graded Sonic hedgehog signalling. Nature 1999; 398:622-627.
74. McDonald JA, Holbrook S, Isshiki T et al. Dorsoventral patterning in the Drosophila central nervous system: the vnd homeobox gene specifies ventral column identity. Genes Dev 1998; 12:3603-3612.
75. Lupo G, Harris WA, Lewis KE. Mechanisms of ventral patterning in the vertebrate nervous system. Nat Rev Neurosci 2006; 7:103-114.
76. Page DT. Inductive patterning of the embryonic brain in Drosophila. Development 2002; 129:2121-2128.
77. Urbach R, Technau GM. Neuroblast formation and patterning during early brain development in Drosophila. BioEssays 2004; 26:739-751.

CHAPTER 4

Dissection of the Embryonic Brain Using Photoactivated Gene Expression

Jonathan Minden*

Abstract

The *Drosophila* brain is generated by a complex series of morphogenetic movements. To better understand brain development and to provide a guide for experimental manipulation of brain progenitors, we created a fate map using photoactivated gene expression to mark cells originating within specific mitotic domains and time-lapse microscopy to dynamically monitor their progeny. We show that mitotic domains 1, 5, 9, 20 and B give rise to discrete cell populations within specific regions of the brain. Mitotic domains 1, 5, 9 and 20 give rise to brain neurons; mitotic domain B produced glial cells. Mitotic domains 5 and 9 produce the antennal and visual sensory systems, respectively, where each sensory system is composed of several disparate cell clusters. Time-lapse analysis of marked cells showed complex mitotic and migratory patterns for cells derived from these mitotic domains.

Introduction

Fate maps serve as critical tools for developmental biologists to chart tissue morphogenesis and as guides for experimental manipulation. The ideal fate map should contain information about cell movements, mitotic patterns, morphology, cell-cell contacts and cell death as well as specific patterns of gene expression and the consequence of altered gene expression and cellular interactions. *Drosophila* fate maps start at the cellular blastoderm stage, which is composed of about 5,000 cells.[1] Prior to this stage there are no lineage-restricted fates, aside from the pole cells.[2] The only physical landmarks at cellular blastoderm are the anterior-posterior and dorsoventral axes. To fate map the embryo, a Cartesian coordinate system relative to percent position along these axes was used to mark the initial position of cells in the blastoderm.[3,4] Mapping was originally done by ablation[4,5] and more recently by dye marking of cells.[6,7] Ablation studies required the removal of rather large numbers of cells since embryos were able to compensate for small losses of cells.[5] The dye marking approaches have been very successful, but are limited in that they do not provide a means to alter the behavior of the marked cells.

Alternative fate mapping methods are: gynandomorph analysis[8] and the generation of mitotic clones.[9] The latter method is useful for producing marked clones of cells. These methods produce genetically perturbed clones of cells, but there is little control over their location.

To develop a more reliable and precise coordinate system than the Cartesian coordinate system, we took advantage of the mitotic domain map. Mitotic domains are bilaterally symmetric groups of cells that divide in a stereotypic sequence that are indicators of cell fate.[10,11] Cells within a mitotic domain are restricted to a limited set of fates that are distinct from the sets of cellular fates observed in neighboring mitotic domains.[12,13]

*Jonathan Minden—Department of Biological Sciences and Science, Carnegie Mellon University, 4400 Fifth Avenue, Pittsburgh, Pennsylvania 15213, USA. Email: minden@cmuedu

Brain Development in Drosophila melanogaster, edited by Gerhard M. Technau.
©2008 Landes Bioscience and Springer Science+Business Media.

To enable the marking of cells in a spatially and temporally restricted manner, we developed a method for activating gene expression using a micro-beam of light.[12] This method, which is referred to as photoactivated gene expression, is based on the GAL4-expression method.[14] Instead of supplying GAL4 genetically, chemically "caged" GAL4VP16 is injected into syncytial stage embryos that carry a UAS-transgene. Expression of the UAS-transgene is activated by briefly irradiating the cell, or cells, of choice with a long-wavelength UV microbeam, thus un-caging the GAL4VP16 protein. This method has been used to activate the expression of benign markers, such as LacZ and GFP, and to alter cell behavior. Time-lapse microscopy and whole-mount embryo preparations are used to track the behavior of marked cells.

This chapter focuses on the origin of the embryonic brain. We show that the brain is derived from five separate mitotic domains, each of which undergo distinct morphogenetic behaviors to generate discrete, non-overlapping regions of the brain. Several different mechanisms are used to internalize blastoderm cells.

Procephalic Blastoderm Fate Map

The procephalic region of the embryo is made up of thirteen mitotic domains (individual mitotic domains will be abbreviated as δN). We have fate mapped eleven procephalic mitotic domains (for δ2, δ8, δ10, δ15 see ref. 12; for δ3, δ18, δ20 see ref. 13; for δ1, δ5, δ9, δB see ref. 15). All of these mitotic domains produced non-overlapping sets of distinctly fated cells. Of these mitotic domains, δ1, δ5, δ9, δ20 and δB form the embryonic brain. We were interested in determining the morphogenetic movements of brain-forming cells. How are these cells internalized? Do they form discrete brain regions? Do they differentiate into neurons and glia? What other cell-types are generated by these mitotic domains? To map the fates of cells within selected mitotic domains, we used photoactivated gene expression to initially mark cells and monitored their development either by three-dimensional, time-lapse microscopy or post-fixation immunohistochemical staining.

Brain-Forming Mitotic Domains Populate Distinct Brain Regions

Mitotic domains 1, 5, 9 and B occupy a large area that roughly corresponds to the procephalic neuroectoderm (Fig. 1A). The strategy for mapping how these mitotic domains contribute to the brain, was to photoactivate patches of cells within a chosen mitotic domain in *UAS-lacZ* or *UAS-nGFP* embryos during stage 8. Photoactivated embryos were aged to stages 14-16 and immuno-stained or live-imaged to detect the expression of the UAS-transgene product. Mitotic domains 1, 5 and 9 generated cells that occupied discrete regions of the brain, suggesting that they may be neurons rather than glial cells, which are scattered.[16] Mitotic domain B produced a dispersed population of cells that will be discussed later. A compendium of many mapping experiments was prepared (Figs. 1B,C and 2B). Each colored line in Figure 1B,C outlines the region of marked cells observed in a single embryo mapped onto a dorsal or lateral view of the embryonic brain. These data show that all three mitotic domains give rise to three distinct, non-overlapping regions of the embryonic brain, demonstrating their early regional specification. The axons emanating from these mitotic domains follow very different paths, indicating their distinct character.

Time-lapse recordings of photoactivated *UAS-nGFP* embryos revealed the complex morphogenetic movements made by each of these mitotic domains to form part of the brain (Fig. 2). The schematic shown in Figure 2B starts at stage 9 when GFP fluorescence is clearly visible, 60-90 minutes following photoactivation. A significant amount of cell movement takes place in the head between stage 7, when cells were photoactivated, and stage 9, placing the cells from each mitotic domain some distance from the site of photoactivation (compare Fig. 1A and Fig 2B, stage 9). The migration pattern is also distinct for each mitotic domain. The following sections will highlight unique features of these mitotic domains.

Mitotic Domain 1 Generates Anterior Protocerebrum Neurons

Mitotic domain 1 is a large, two-lobed region. Photoactivation of different regions of δ1 generated clones of different cell-types. Photoactivation of the anterior-ventral region of δ1 revealed that

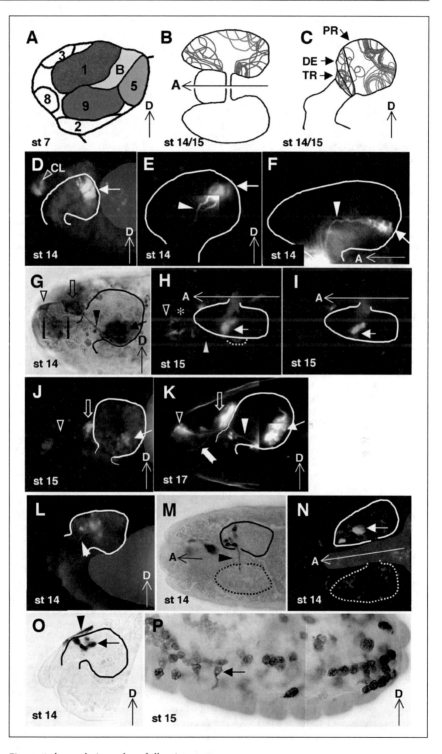

Figure 1, legend viewed on following page.

Figure 1, viewed on previous page. Fate mapping of δ1, δ5, and δ9 cells. For all figures, the embryo anterior is to the left. Dorsally mounted embryos are indicated by a horizontal arrow pointing to the anterior, marked A. Laterally mounted embryos are indicated by a vertical arrow pointing dorsally, marked D. The stage of the embryo is indicated in the bottom left corner of each panel. A) Schematic representation of the head mitotic domains at stage 7, which was used to guide photoactivation experiments. B,C) Cartoon of the regions within the embryonic brain that are populated by each mitotic domain. Each line represents results from an individual embryo (δ1-red n = 31, δ5-green n = 21, δ9-blue n = 31). The remaining panels show micrographs of photoactivated embryos. The affected brain hemisphere is bounded by a solid line. D-F) Photoactivation of δ1. D) 2-4 cell photoactivation of a *UAS-nGFP* embryo stained with anti-GFP antibody (green) and anti-ELAV (red). The δ1 derived cells are visible in both the brain (solid arrow) and the clypeolabrum (CL). E,F) 2-4 cell photoactivation of *UAS-tauGFP* embryos. The arrowheads indicate the pioneer axons of the embryonic peduncle. G-K) Photoactivation of δ5. All images are of 5-8 cell photoactivations. G) A photoactivated *UAS-lacZ* embryo showing the four different δ5 structures: the posterior group within the brain (solid arrow), the middle group just anterior to the brain (open arrow), the anterior group (open arrowhead) and the epithelial group (bracketed). The axon connecting the posterior and middle groups is indicated by the closed arrowhead. H,I) A *UAS-lacZ* embryo stained with antibodies against β-galactosidase (green) and FasII (red). H) Composite image of 3 adjacent optical sections showing FasII-positive: optic lobe (outlined with dashed line), Bolwig's organ (asterisk) and Bolwig's nerve (yellow arrowhead). GFP-expressing, δ5 brain cells are in a different focal plane (solid arrow) that is adjacent to optic lobe. The δ5 anterior group (open arrowhead) is adjacent to Bolwig's organ. I) An in-focus optical section of the GFP-positive δ5 cells within the brain (solid arrow). J) A δ5 photoactivated *UAS-nGFP* embryo stained with anti-GFP (green) and anti-ELAV (red; using the same arrow scheme as panel G). K) Composite of projected images of a δ5-photoactivated, *UAS-tauGFP* embryo (using the same arrow scheme as panel G). The bifurcated axon tract projecting to the maxillary complex is indicated by a notched arrow. L-P) Photoactivation of δ9. L) 2-4 cell photoactivation of a *UAS-lacZ* embryo stained with anti-β–galactosidase (green) and anti-ELAV (red). The closed arrowhead indicates an axon extending toward the ventral nerve cord. M) Single cell photoactivation of a *UAS-lacZ* embryo histochemically stained with anti-β–galactosidase. The closed arrowhead indicates an axon extending to contralateral brain hemisphere. N) 2-4 cell photoactivation of a *UAS-lacZ* embryo stained with anti-β–galactosidase (green) and anti-Repo (red). The arrow indicates the patch of β-galactosidase-positive cells that were not expressing Repo. O) Single cell photoactivation of δ9 in a *UAS-lacZ* embryo histochemically stained with anti-β–galactosidase showing marked epidermal (closed arrowhead) and brain cells (closed arrow). P) 5-8 cell photoactivation of δ9 in a *UAS-lacZ* embryo histochemically stained with anti-β–galactosidase showing marked migratory cells (arrow) throughout the entire embryo. Yolk auto-fluorescence which appears in the green fluorescence channel is masked gray in D, J, L and N. Reprinted from: Robertson K et al. Dev Biol 2003; 260:124-137; ©2003 with permission from Elsevier.[15]

this region contributed mostly to the clypeolabrum (Fig. 1D, see the green fluorescent cells outside of the brain as indicated by the letters CL). The posterior-dorsal region gave rise to cells located predominantly in the anterior-medial part of the protocerebrum (when referring to brain location, we use the neuroaxis as the frame of reference) (Fig. 1D-F and cartooned in Fig. 1B,C, see the areas bounded by the red lines). These results indicate that δ1 is divided into two sub-regions.

In the protocerebrum, marked δ1 cells populated two adjacent clusters of cells. These cells co-labeled with the pan-neuronal marker, ELAV (Fig. 1D, arrow).[17] In contrast, very few δ1-derived cells expressed the glial cell marker, Repo.[18] Less than 2% of the marked δ1 cells were glia, indicating that δ1 cells gave rise to neurons rather than bipotential progenitors. Time-lapse analysis of photoactivated δ1 cells showed that these cells were internalized *en mass*. The mass then moved posteriorly along the midline to their final position in the protocerebrum (Fig. 2B).

The location and double cluster appearance of δ1 neurons suggested that they may form the embryonic mushroom bodies. To further test this possibility, δ1 axons were marked by photoactivation using *UAS-tauGFP* embryos. These TauGFP marked axons had the typical morphology of the embryonic mushroom bodies (Fig. 1E,F, arrowhead).[19,20]

Mitotic Domain 5 Produces the Embryonic Antennal System

Mitotic domain 5, which is initially located just anterior to the cephalic furrow near the dorsal midline (Fig. 1A), produces four distinct cell populations; one epidermal and three neuronal (Fig. 1G, 2A,B). Time-lapse analysis of photoactivated *UAS-nGFP* embryos revealed the complex migration pattern of this mitotic domain (Fig. 2A). The photoactivated patch of cells first elongated along the edge of the cephalic furrow adjacent to the maxillary segment (Fig. 2A, frame 1, stage 9). The most anterior-ventral cells remained in the epidermis and moved to the anterior tip of the embryo. As head involution began, the non-epidermal δ5 progeny became internalized at the boundary between the mandibulary and maxillary segments and separated into two populations (Fig. 2A, frames 5-6, stages 13-14). The inward movement of these cells appeared to be via invagination. One population, the posterior group, which ultimately forms the antennal lobe of the brain, remained stationary at the mid-anterior region of the embryonic brain, while the second group migrated over the ventral surface of the developing brain (Fig. 2A, frames 6-7, stage 14-15). This was followed by another splitting of cells from the second group, which migrated into the position of the antennal sensory organ (Fig. 2A, frames 7, stage 15). This culminated in populations of ~20 posterior group, ~5-6 middle group and 2-4 anterior group cells; the number of epidermal cells was not determined.

Immuno-chemical staining of δ5 photoactivated *UAS-lacZ* embryos showed that the three internalized populations were connected by axonal fibers (Fig. 1G, solid arrowhead). All four groups of cells arising from δ5 are shown in Fig. 1G. The neuronal character of cells within these groups was revealed by counter-staining with anti-ELAV antibody; about half of the photoactivated cells within the anterior and posterior groups expressed ELAV (Fig. 1J, arrow, open arrowhead). We further confirmed the neuronal nature of the δ5 derived brain cells, as well as those of the anterior group, by photoactivating δ5 cells in *UAS-tauGFP* embryos. Tau-GFP highlighted the axons of the posterior group within the brain, the axon tracts between the groups and the structure of the most anterior group (Fig. 1K). The axons of the δ5-derived brain cells can also be seen extending into other parts of the brain (Fig. 1K). Many of these processes appear to terminate in the region of the brain populated by δ1 mushroom body precursors (compare Fig. 1K and E, which correspond to δ5 and δ1, respectively).

The pattern of δ5 cell types was reminiscent of the cell types produced by δ20, which will be described later.[13] The morphogenetic movements of δ5 and δ20 were also similar; but not identical, δ20 cells form a more elongated pattern prior to internalization. We confirmed that mitotic domains 5 and 20 yielded different structures by photoactivating δ5 cells in *UAS-lacZ* embryos and immuno-stained for FasII and β-galactosidase expression. FasII is expressed in the optic lobe, Bolwig's nerve and Bolwig's organ, but not antennal cells.[21] FasII was not expressed in any of the photoactivated δ5 cells (Fig. 1H,I). δ5-derived brain cells (Fig. 1H,I, closed arrow) were adjacent to the optic lobe (Fig. 1H and I, broken line); there was no overlap. Likewise, δ5 cells in the anterior group (Fig. 1H, open arrowhead) were adjacent to Bolwig's organ, not overlapping (Fig. 1H, asterisk). Thus, δ5-derived cells do not contribute to any part of the visual system.

The morphology and position of the δ5-derived cells indicate that this mitotic domain gives rise to the antennal sensory system, where the anterior group corresponds to the antennal sensory organ and the posterior group, which is in the brain, corresponds to the antennal lobe.

Mitotic Domain 9 Produces Three Apparently Unrelated Cell Types

A unique feature of δ9 is that the entire cell population divides perpendicularly to the embryonic surface during the 14th mitosis, creating two populations of cells, predicted to be epidermal and brain.[10] To ensure that both layers of progeny were marked, δ9 cells were irradiated prior to, or during, the 14th mitosis. Three distinct cell types were derived from δ9: posterior brain (Fig. 1L-N), dorsal midline epidermis (Fig. 1O, closed arrowhead) and an unidentified population of migratory cells (Fig. 1P).

To determine the lineage relationship of these three cell populations, different-sized patches of cells within δ9 were photoactivated in *UAS-lacZ* and *UAS-GFP* embryos (Table 1). Time-lapse

Table 1. Distribution of different cell types arising from δ9

Cell Type(s)*	Single Cell Photoactivation (Percent, n = 29)	2-4 Cell Photoactivation (Percent, n = 72)	5-8 Cell Photoactivation (Percent, n = 24)
E	10	4	0
B	31	15	0
M	7	21	12
E + B	45	13	13
E + M	0	0	0
B + M	0	28	29
E + B + M	7	19	46

*E indicates epithelial cells; B indicates brain cells; M indicates migratory cells. Different sized patches of δ9 cells were photoactivated in *UAS-lacZ* embryos just prior to, or during, the 14th mitosis. The embryos were aged to stage 14 through 16 and stained with anti-β-galactosidase antibody. Only embryos with multiple marked cells were scored. Reprinted from: Robertson K et al. Dev Biol 2003; 260:124-137; ©2003 with permission from Elsevier.[15]

recordings showed that all three cell types experienced significant amounts of cell death, making it extremely difficult to draw firm conclusions about lineage relationships. The origin of the migratory cells is not clear. None of the clones were composed of both epithelial and migratory cells, indicating that epithelial cells do not give rise to migratory cells directly. Thus, the migratory cells are either derived from brain progenitors or delaminated directly from the blastoderm. A significant fraction of embryos had marked migratory-only clones, particularly with 2-4 cell photoactivation, supporting the delamination hypothesis. The brain- and migratory-cell progenitors appear to be evenly distributed across δ9.

Time-lapse analysis revealed that initially the brain and epidermal progenitors moved in unison anterior and dorsally, before separating, leaving the epidermal cells at the dorsal midline (Fig. 2B, stage 12, blue hatching), while the brain progenitors continue to move posteriorly to their final location in the brain (Fig. 2B). All photoactivated δ9 brain cells expressed ELAV (Fig. 1L); none expressed Repo (Fig. 1N), indicating δ9-derived brain cells are neurons, not glia. These neurons occupied the deutero-, proto- and tritocerebrum (Fig. 1C,L), thus, the formation of the three cerebral neuromeres does not appear to be specified by separate mitotic domains. In many embryos an axon could be seen to project either through the tritocerebrum toward the ventral nerve cord (Fig. 1L, closed arrowhead) or toward the contralateral hemisphere through the tritocerebral commissure (Fig. 1M, closed arrowhead). These structures are similar to those described by Therianos et al.[22]

Mitotic Domain 20 Generates the Entire Visual System

Mitotic domain 20 is the most posterior of the three dorsal head mitotic domains (Fig. 3A). A small number of cells within δ20 was marked by photoactivating *UAS-lacZ* expression. Since the cells in δ20 divide much later than surrounding mitotic domains and most of the cells divide inside the cephalic furrow,[10] it was difficult to distinguish δ20 cells as they divide. Therefore, δ20 cells were identified as those cells surrounded by the amnioserosa and mitotic domains 5, 18 and B (Fig. 3A, green circle).

Photoactivating cells in the center of δ20 gave rise to a set of bilaterally symmetrical structures spanning from the anterior tip to the brain (Fig. 3B), including many head sensory organs and nerves of the peripheral nervous system (PNS), the posterior part of the brain, and the dorsal pouch epithelium above the clypeolabrum. Activation of δ20 cells also gave rise to a significant amount of cellular debris, indicating that some cells were dying. Photoactivation procedure does not affect cell death patterns.[12]

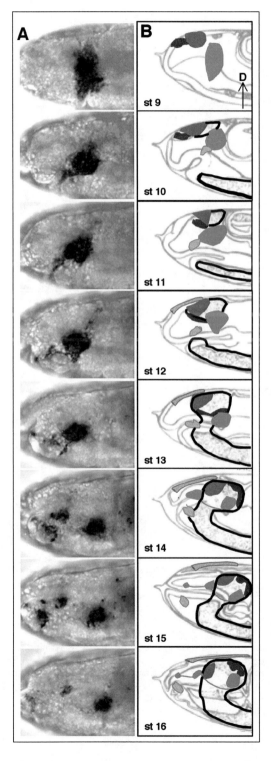

Figure 2. Time-lapse images and cartoon of *UAS-nGFP* embryo following photoactivation. Column A) A series of images from a time-lapse recording of a δ5 photoactivated embryo. The GFP fluorescence is shown in negative so that marked cells appear black overlaying transmitted light images. Lateral view of stages 9-16 as a projection of seven 5 μm optical sections. Column B) Diagrammatic representation of the position of the progeny from mitotic domains 1, 5, and 9 from stage 9 to 16 shown as a lateral view. This series was constructed from multiple time-lapse experiments (δ1-red, δ5-green, δ9-blue, the brain is outlined in black). Reprinted from: Robertson K et al. Dev Biol 2003; 260:124-137; ©2003 with permission from Elsevier.[15]

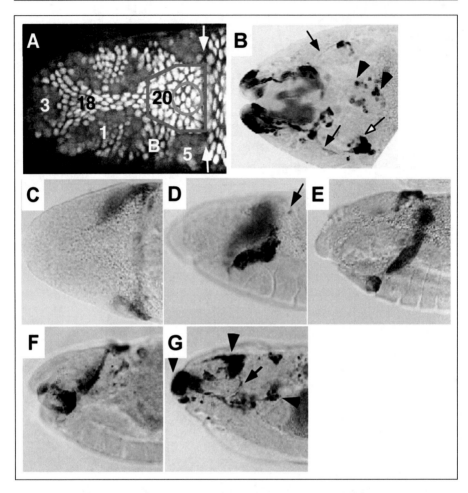

Figure 3. Fate mapping of δ20. A) Individual cells of the dorsal head mitotic domains were visualized by the expression of nuclear GFP (*Ubi-GFPnls*) by confocal microscopy. δ20 is highlighted with a gray border. The numbers indicate mitotic domains. Interphase nuclei appear bright and have sharp edges while mitotic cells are large and appear diffuse. The white arrows point to the cephalic furrow. The gray circle indicates a typical size and location of the UV photoactivation beam. All embryos are shown with anterior to the left. B) Fates of mitotic domains were visualized by GAL4 dependent activation of *lacZ* using the photoactivated gene expression system. Shown here is a dorsal view of a stage 17 embryo with photoactivated δ20 cells. Cells in the posterior part of the brain (white arrow) and head PNS (including axons projecting to the brain; arrows) were marked as well as cellular debris (arrow heads). C-G) Developmental time-course of δ20. Dorsal (C) and lateral (D to G) images of δ20-photoactivated embryos. The marked cells were visualized with an anti-β-galactosidase antibody. C) The cells in δ20 moved away from the dorsal midline during germband extension. D) At late stage 11, the cells reached the dorsal border of the gnathal segments. The first sign of cell death was apparent as a small spot moving away from the group of marked cells (arrow). E) At stage 13, the marked δ20 cells extended along the lateral surface. F) During stage 14, the ventral cells continued to move anteriorly into the stomodeal invagination. G) At the end of embryogenesis, cells were distributed into three clusters (arrowheads); the anterior tip, dorsal pouch and the brain, connected via nerve-like projections (arrow). Reprinted from: Namba R, Minden JS. Dev Biol 1999; 212:465-476; ©1999 with permission from Elsevier.[13]

δ20 starts as a single domain on the dorsal midline. During germband extension, the cells of δ20 moved bilaterally away from the dorsal midline (Fig. 3C). By two hours after photoactivation at stage 7, most δ20 cells had migrated laterally away from the dorsal midline where they formed the dorsal border of the gnathal segments (Fig. 3D). By the end of stage 13, the cells formed a narrow strip spanning from the ventral to the dorsal surface (Fig. 3E). At the end of embryogenesis, cells in this narrow strip were distributed into three clusters spanning the entire length of the head (Fig. 3F). The ventral δ20 cells moved anteriorly with the gnathal segments during stomodeal invagination (Fig. 3G) and eventually reached the anterior tip. The more dorsal δ20 cells formed the dorsal ridge and became a part of the dorsal pouch, while some cells delaminated and occupied the ventral posterior part of the brain lobe. The cells in the brain lobe were usually connected to a cell cluster in the anterior tip of the embryo by long nerve-like projections (Fig. 3G arrow).

Photoactivation of δ20 marked a pair of lateral clusters of cells in the dorsal pouch adjacent to the pharynx in the stage 16 embryo (Fig. 4A). This cluster projected a nerve to the posterior part of the brain and the entire projection path was marked by the *lacZ* expression. The location and morphology of this structure suggested that it was the larval photoreceptor organ, Bolwig's organ, which was confirmed by staining with a PNS-specific antibody, mAb 22C10.[23,24] Double staining δ20 activated embryos for β-galactosidase expression and with mAb22C10 showed that the photoactivated δ20 cells coincided with the Bolwig's organ, fasciculated axons of the Bolwig's organ (Bolwig's nerve), and cells at the termini of Bolwig's nerve presumably in the optic lobe (Fig. 4B).

In addition to producing the larval visual system, some δ20 cells were observed to form an epithelium on top of the Bolwig's nerve projection path (Fig. 4, white arrows). The Bolwig's nerve

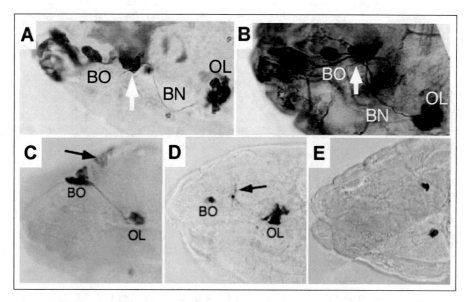

Figure 4. δ20 generates the larval visual system. A,B) Dorsal view of δ20 marked embryos. A) β-galactosidase was expressed in the Bolwig's organ (BO), Bolwig's nerve (BN) and the optic lobe (OL). White arrows point to cells in the dorsal pouch on top of the Bolwig's nerve path. B) β-galactosidase expression (blue) in the larval visual system overlaps with PNS marker expression as visualized with mAb22C10 (brown). C-E) Single-cell photoactivation of δ20; marked cells were found in the developing larval visual system at stage 14 (C) and at stage 17 (D), both lateral views. They were confined to the Bolwig's organ (BO), the optic lobe (OL) and the dorsal pouch (arrows). E) A dorsal view of an embryo with marked cells in both optic lobes. Reprinted from: Namba R, Minden JS. Dev Biol 1999; 212:465-476; ©1999 with permission from Elsevier.[13] A color version of this figure is available online at www.eurekah.com.

extends posteriorly from the Bolwig's organ located inside the dorsal pouch epithelium and makes a sharp, ventral turn near the posterior edge of the dorsal pouch to follow along the basal surface of the brain into the optic lobe. The δ20 cells that formed the epithelial structure were often found at or near where the Bolwig's nerve made the ventral turn, which corresponds to the location of the eye-antennal disc placode.

Photoactivation of single cells in the center of δ20 gave rise to marked cells in the optic lobe, Bolwig's organ, and a small area of the dorsal pouch, presumably the eye-antennal disc placode, exclusively (Fig. 4C,D). This photoactivation typically marked the larval visual system either on the left- or right-hand side of the embryo, while a small fraction of these embryos had marked, visual system cells on both sides of the embryo midline (Fig. 4E). These results show that all of the cell-types that make up the larval visual system can be derived from a single δ20 cell.

Mitotic Domain B Generates Brain Glia

Progeny of mitotic domains 1, 5 and 9 populated almost all of the brain volume (Fig. 1B,C). None of these mitotic domains generated significant numbers of glial cells. Photoactivation of the remaining mitotic domain, δB, revealed a major source of brain glia. Photoactivation of cells in three locations along the length of this elongated mitotic domain (Fig. 1A) in *UAS-nGFP* embryos revealed that their progeny formed small clusters of cells in the presumptive protocerebrum at stage 14 (Fig. 5A, solid arrow). The distribution of these clusters in the stage 14 embryonic brain is diagrammed in Figure 5E,F. These clusters were located deep within the brain and were variable in size. Each of the clusters of marked δB cells was surrounded by dispersed cells (Fig. 5A and cartooned as dots in

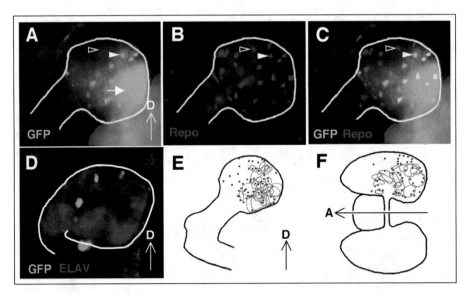

Figure 5. Brain glia originate from δB. A-C) 2-4 cell photoactivation of δB in a *UAS-nGFP* embryo stained with anti-GFP (green) and anti-Repo (red). A) Shows the green fluorescent channel. A cluster of GFP-positive cells below the focal plane (indicated by the solid arrow) that is surrounded by individual cells (solid arrowhead). B) Shows the anti-Repo signal revealing glial cells. C) Shows the superposition of A and B. Notice the double labeled cells (solid arrowhead) and Repo-only glial cells (open arrowhead). D) 2-4 cell photoactivation of δB in a *UAS-nGFP* embryo stained with anti-GFP (green) and anti-ELAV (red). Notice that none of the GFP-positive cells also express the neuronal marker, ELAV. E,F) Schematic representations of marked δB cells within the brain, lateral and dorsal views, respectively. The blue outlined areas represent marked clusters; the blue dots represent isolated cells. Reprinted from: Robertson K et al. Dev Biol 2003; 260:124-137; ©2003 with permission from Elsevier.[15]

Fig. 5E,F). Three-quarters of δB photoactivated embryos had marked, dispersed brain cells that also expressed Repo, indicating that they were glial cells (Fig. 5A-C). None of the marked cells in δB photoactivated embryos expressed ELAV (Fig. 5D), indicating that they are unlikely to be neurons. There are two classes of embryonic brain glia: the subperineural glia that are mostly located in the brain periphery and the neuropil glia.[16] Glial cells arising from δB were identified as subperineural glia by their position. Neuropil glia were never observed, suggesting that this subtype of glial cells may arise from a different source.

Conclusion

The most difficult aspect of fate mapping the head region of the *Drosophila* embryo is its complex morphogenesis. We have fate mapped the majority of mitotic domains within the *Drosophila* procephalic blastoderm using the photoactivated gene expression system and determined that the embryonic brain develops from five mitotic domains: δ1 (posterior-dorsal part), δ5, δ9, δ20 and δB. The final position of the mitotic domain progeny within the brain does not reflect their relative blastoderm positions. Thus, the mitotic domains follow specific morphogenetic trajectories. Several different mechanisms are employed to internalize brain progenitors: the posterior-dorsal part of δ1 and δB invaginate en mass, δ5 and δ20 also invaginate together, and δ9 uses oriented mitosis and possibly delamination. Together, these mitotic domains constitute non-overlapping regions of the brain. This fate map will provide an avenue for performing region-specific experiments. The discrete behavior of the brain-forming mitotic domains raises several interesting questions about the ancestral origin of the brain. One such question is, did the various brain compartments evolve from a common group of cells and later specialize or did the compartments evolve independently and later coalesce to form the brain?

References

1. Foe VE, Odell GM, Edgar BA. Mitosis and morphogenesis in the Drosophila embryo. In: Bate M, Martinez AA, eds. The Development of Drosophila melanogaster. New York: Cold Spring Harbor Laboratory Press, 1993:149-300.
2. St. Johnston D. Pole plasm and the posterior group genes. In: Bate M, Martinez AA, eds. The Development of Drosophila melanogaster. New York: Cold Spring Harbor Laboratory Press, 1993:325-364.
3. Hartenstein V, Technau GM, Campos-Ortega JA. Fate-mapping in wild-type Drosophila melanogaster. III. A fate map of the blastoderm. Roux's Arch Dev Biol 1985; 194:213-216.
4. Jurgens GR, Lehman M, Schardin M et al. Segmental organization of the head in the embryo of Drosophila melanogaster. A blastoderm fate map of the cuticle structures of the larval head. Roux's Arch Dev Biol 1986; 195:359-377.
5. Underwood EM, Turner FR, Mahowald AP. Analysis of cell movements and fate mapping during early embryogenesis in Drosophila melanogaster. Dev Biol 1980; 74(2):286-301.
6. Bossing T, Technau GM. The fate of the CNS midline progenitors in Drosophila as revealed by a new method for single cell labelling. Development 1994; 120(7):1895-1906.
7. Technau GM, Campos-Ortega JA. Fate-mapping in wild-type Drosophila. II. Injections of horseradish peroxidase in cells of the early gastrula stage. Roux's Arch Dev Biol 1985; 194:196-212.
8. Gehring WJ, Wieschaus E, Holliger M. The use of 'normal' and 'transformed' gynandromorphs in mapping the primordial germ cells and the gonadal mesoderm in Drosophila. J Embryol Exp Morphol 1976; 35(3):607-616.
9. Janning W. Aldehyde oxidase as a cell marker for internal organs in Drosophila melanogaster. Naturwissenschaften 1972; 59(11):516-517.
10. Foe VE. Mitotic domains reveal early commitment of cells in Drosophila embryos. Development 1989; 107(1):1-22.
11. Minden JS, Agard DA, Sedat JW, et al. Direct cell lineage analysis in Drosophila melanogaster by time-lapse, three-dimensional optical microscopy of living embryos. J Cell Biol 1989; 109(2):505-516.
12. Cambridge SB, Davis RL, Minden JS. Drosophila mitotic domain boundaries as cell fate boundaries. Science 1997; 277(5327):825-828.
13. Namba R, Minden JS. Fate mapping of Drosophila embryonic mitotic domain 20 reveals that the larval visual system is derived from a subdomain of a few cells. Dev Biol 1999; 212(2):465-476.
14. Brand AH, Perrimon N. Targeted gene expression as a means of altering cell fates and generating dominant phenotypes. Development 1993; 118(2):401-415.

15. Robertson K, Mergliano J, Minden JS. Dissecting Drosophila embryonic brain development using photoactivated gene expression. Dev Biol 2003; 260(1):124-137.
16. Hartenstein V, Nassif C, Lekven A. Embryonic development of the Drosophila brain. II. Pattern of glial cells. J Comp Neurol 1998; 402(1):32-47.
17. Koushika SP, Lisbin MJ, White K. ELAV, a Drosophila neuron-specific protein, mediates the generation of an alternatively spliced neural protein isoform. Curr Biol 1996; 6(12):1634-1641.
18. Halter DA, Urban J, Rickert C et al. The homeobox gene repo is required for the differentiation and maintenance of glia function in the embryonic nervous system of Drosophila melanogaster. Development 1995; 121(2):317-332.
19. Tettamanti M, Armstrong, DJ, Endo K et al. Early development of the Drosophila mushroom bodies, brain centers for associative learning and memory. Dev Genes Evol 1997; 207:242-252.
20. Kurusu M, Awasaki T, Masuda-Nakagawa LM et al. Embryonic and larval development of the Drosophila mushroom bodies: concentric layer subdivisions and the role of fasciclin II. Development 2002; 129(2):409-419.
21. Holmes AL, Heilig JS. Fasciclin II and Beaten path modulate intercellular adhesion in Drosophila larval visual organ development. Development 1999; 126(2):261-272.
22. Therianos S, Leuzinger S, Hirth F et al. Embryonic development of the Drosophila brain: formation of commissural and descending pathways. Development 1995; 121(11):3849-3860.
23. Fujita SC, Zipursky SL, Benzer S et al. Monoclonal antibodies against the Drosophila nervous system. Proc Natl Acad Sci USA 1982; 79(24):7929-7933.
24. Goodman CS, Bastiani MJ, Doe CQ et al. Cell recognition during neuronal development. Science 1984; 225(4668):1271-1279.

CHAPTER 5

Design of the Larval Chemosensory System

Reinhard F. Stocker*

Abstract

Given that smell and taste are vital senses for most animal species, it is not surprising that chemosensation has become a strong focus in neurobiological research. Much of what we know today about how the brain "mirrors" the chemical environment has derived from simple organisms like *Drosophila*. This is because their chemosensory system includes only a fraction of the cell number of the mammalian system, yet often exhibits the same basic design. Recent studies aimed at establishing fruitfly larvae as a particularly simple model for smell and taste have analyzed the expression patterns of olfactory and gustatory receptors, the circuitry of the chemosensory system and its behavioral output. Surprisingly, the larval olfactory system shares the organization of its adult counterpart, though comprising much reduced cell numbers. It thus indeed provides a "minimal" model system of general importance. Comparing adult and larval chemosensory systems raises interesting questions about their functional capabilities and about the processes underlying its transformation through metamorphosis.

Introduction

The senses of smell and taste create representations of the chemical environment in the brain. Understanding how the nervous system fulfills this amazing task—given the diversity of molecules, concentrations and blends—is a major challenge in neurobiology. A breakthrough in chemosensory research was prompted by the identification of odorant receptor genes in rodents,[1] in *C. elegans*,[2] and in *Drosophila*.[3,4] The expression patterns of these genes turned out to be an ideal tool for dissecting the olfactory circuits.[5-8] These studies allowed to confirm earlier assumptions that the olfactory systems of mammals and insects are organized according to common principles,[9-11] even though the insect brain comprises only a fraction of the cell numbers of the mammalian brain. It is therefore not surprising that insect species like *Manduca sexta, Apis mellifera* and *D. melanogaster* have become attractive models for investigating the chemical senses.

Does the larval chemosensory system of flies or other holometabolous insects offer an even simpler alternative? Adults and larvae are anatomically and behaviorally much different, reflecting their different life-styles. Adult flies, for example, search for food, mates, and egg-laying substrates, all of which requires sophisticated odor analysis. Fly larvae, in contrast, live directly on their food, and hence may not need long-range odor detection. Compatible with this notion, their olfactory system in terms of cell numbers is massively reduced. Nevertheless, its basic organization is surprisingly similar to the adult design, turning the *Drosophila* larva into a new, "elementary" model system for smell.[12-15]

*Dr. Reinhard F. Stocker—Department of Biology, University of Fribourg,10, Chemin du Musée, CH-1700 Fribourg, Switzerland. Email: reinhard.stocker@unifr.ch

Brain Development in Drosophila melanogaster, edited by Gerhard M. Technau.
©2008 Landes Bioscience and Springer Science+Business Media.

Chemosensory Organs of the Larval Head

The chemosensory equipment of the larval head of *D. melanogaster* includes three external sense organs, dorsal organ (DO), terminal organ (TO) and ventral organ (VO), as well as three pharyngeal organs[16-21] (Fig. 1). Each of these organs consists of several sensilla comprising one to nine neurons and three accessory cells, all of which are collected below a common cuticular hair or terminal pore. The DO is composed of a multiporous "dome" suggesting olfactory function, as well as six peripheral sensilla. In *Musca*, five of these six peripheral sensilla and most of the TO and VO sensilla are characterized by a terminal pore indicating gustatory function.[22-24] In *Drosophila*, the olfactory function of the dome was confirmed by electrophysiological recording[13,25] and genetic ablation studies.[12,26,27] Indeed, selective block of the 21 sensory neurons of the dome confirmed their identity as the unique odorant receptor neurons (ORNs) of the larva.[12,27] Hence, the DO seems to be a mixed organ for smell and taste, while the TO and the VO respond to tastants only. In addition, all three organs may also include mechanosensory,[22-24] thermosensory,[28] and hygrosensory neurons. The ganglia of the DO, TO and VO comprise 36-37, 32 and 7 sensory neurons, respectively.[20] The dendrites of the 21 ORNs of the DO extend as seven triplets into the dome, 12 additional DO neurons innervate the six peripheral sensilla of the DO, and the remaining three DO neurons atypically project toward one of the TO sensilla.[20,29,30]

The dorsal and ventral pharyngeal sense organs comprising 17 and 16 neurons, respectively, are situated immediately behind the mouthhooks. They include multiple sensilla and may represent gustatory and mechanosensory organs.[16,20,21] The small posterior pharyngeal sense organ is located further back on the gut and is composed of two sensilla with three neurons each.[21]

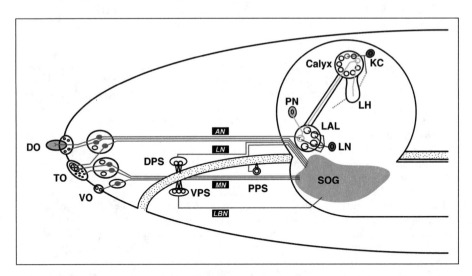

Figure 1. The chemosensory system of the larval head. The dorsal organ (DO) comprises the olfactory dome (grey) and a few putative taste sensilla (small circles). The terminal organ (TO), the ventral organ (VO), as well as the dorsal, ventral and posterior pharyngeal sense organs (DPS, VPS and PPS, respectively) include mainly taste sensilla. Neuronal cell bodies are collected in ganglia below each sense organ. Three neurons innervating the TO are located in the ganglion of the DO. Odorant receptor neurons (blue) from the dome send their axon via the antennal nerve *(AN)* into the larval antennal lobe (LAL). Local interneurons (LN) interconnect the glomeruli of the LAL, while projection neurons (PN; green) link the LAL with the mushroom body calyx and the lateral horn (LH). An intrinsic mushroom body Kenyon cell (KC; red) is shown. Axons from putative taste receptor neurons (brown) extend via four different nerves to the CNS and end in the suboesophageal region (SOG). *LBN* labial nerve, *LN* labral nerve, *MN* maxillary nerve.

Olfactory projections in the CNS are supra-oesophageal, whereas taste information is sent to the sub-oesophageal ganglion (Fig. 1). Different from adults, all olfactory projections remain ipsilateral. Neurons from the DO ganglion, regardless of their modality and irrespective of whether they extend to the DO or TO, connect to the brain via the antennal nerve.[20,31] The supra-oesophageal labral nerve carries the afferents from the dorsal and posterior pharyngeal sense organs, whereas the sub-oesophageal maxillary and labial nerves comprise those from the TO and VO ganglia, and from the ventral pharyngeal sense organ, respectively.[17,18,20,21]

Olfactory System

Odorant Receptors and Their Expression Patterns

Odorant receptors (ORs) define the spectrum of detectable odors. Their expression pattern across the population of ORNs provides the basis for a combinatorial code in their target areas in the brain which allows to interpret a practically unlimited number of odors and odor mixtures. This seems to be true both for mammals[1,5,6] and for *Drosophila*.[3,4,7,8]

In adult *Drosophila*, two related sub-families of chemosensory receptors have been identified, an OR family comprising 62 members[3,4,32,33] and a family of gustatory receptors (GRs) with 60 members (see *Gustatory Receptors and Their Expression Pattern*).[32-36] Similar to mammals, fly ORNs express in general a single OR.[3,4,37,38] For many ORs, odorant response spectra and expression patterns have been studied.[37,39] Afferents of ORNs expressing a given OR converge onto one or two glomeruli in the antennal lobe,[7,8,40] analogous to the mammalian olfactory system. Hence, odor information carried by ORNs is translated into a pattern of glomerular activation.[41-44]

The logic of *Or* gene expression in the larval olfactory system, despite its simplicity, is surprisingly similar to the adult logic.[12,13,27] For 25 *Or* genes, expression was shown by in situ hybridization and via *Or-Gal4* driver lines (Table 1).[12] However, there is evidence of a few additional candidate larval *Or* genes.[12,13,45] Each of the 21 larval ORNs expresses the atypical receptor OR83b, known also from adult flies, which is involved in proper localization and function of "conventional" ORs.[27,46,47] The large majority of the ORNs express one conventional OR along with OR83b, while two ORNs were shown to coexpress two additional ORs apart from OR83b.[12] Given that the number of identified ORs exceeds the total number of ORNs, a few more cases of triple OR expression are to be expected. Taken together, the number of primary olfactory "qualities" in the larva, reflected by the number of ORs expressed, is considerably smaller compared to the approximately 60 qualities in adults. Interestingly, of the 25 well characterized larval *Or* genes, 13 are larval-specific,[12,13] whereas the remaining 12 *Or* genes are expressed in adults as well (Table 1).[3,4,8,32,48]

Using the "emtpy neuron approach", i.e., expressing single *Or* genes in adult anosmic mutant ORNs,[37-39] the electrophysiological responses of 11 larval ORs to a panel of 29 known adult or larval stimulants[26,38,39,49-51] were recorded.[13] The reaction spectra observed were very diverse, ranging from an OR that responded only to a single tested odorant, to ORs which responded up to nine odorants.[13] Odorants that elicited strong responses usually did so from multiple receptors. Some ORs responded most strongly to aliphatic compounds, while others were preferentially tuned to aromatic compounds. Most of the responses were excitatory, but some ORs were strongly inhibited by one compound and excited by another. Response dynamics and odor sensitivities varied largely among different receptors.

Glomerular Architecture of the Larval Antennal Lobe

The larval olfactory circuitry is surprisingly similar to the adult circuitry, though much reduced in terms of cell numbers. Olfactory afferents terminate in the larval antennal lobe (LAL). Their targets are local interneurons, which provide lateral connections in the LAL, and projection neurons (PNs), which link the LAL via the inner antennocerebral tract with higher order olfactory centers, the mushroom body (MB) calyx and the lateral horn (Fig. 1).[15,20,52] Analogous to the adult fly, larval ORNs and PNs seem to be cholinergic, whereas most or even all of the local interneurons may be GABAergic.[53]

Table 1. OR genes and GR genes expressed in the larva

		In Situ Hybridization	Gal4 Driver Lines
Or1a	L	+	+
Or2a	L + A	+	
Or7a	L + A	+	
Or13a	L + A	+	+
Or22a	*L + A*		+
Or22c	L	+	+
Or24a	L	+	+
Or30a	L	+	+
Or33a	L + A	+	+
Or33b*	L + A	+	+
Or35a	L + A	+	+
Or42a	L + A	+	+
Or42b	L + A	+	+
Or45a	L	+	+
Or45b	L	+	+
Or47a*	L + A	+	+
Or49a	L + A		+
Or59a	L	+	+
Or63a	L	+	+
Or67b	L + A	+	+
Or67c	*L + A*		+
Or74a	L	+	+
Or82a	L + A	+	+
Or83a	L	+	+
Or83b***	L + A	+	+
Or85c	L	+	
Or85d	*L + A*		+
Or94a**	L	+	
Or94b**	L	+	
Gr2a	L + A		+
Gr21a	L + A		+
Gr22e	L + A		+
Gr28be	L + A		+
Gr32a	L + A		+
Gr63a	L + A		+
Gr66a	L + A		+

L/A: expression in larval/adult chemosensory neurons. Or33b/Or47a (*) and Or94a/Or94b (**) are coexpressed in the same ORN.[12] Or83b (***) encodes an atypical, ubiquitously expressed OR.[12,27] Or data are from references 12 and 13, data in *italics* from reference 45, and Gr data are from references 12 and 36.

The expression patterns of ORN-specific *Gal4* driver lines revealed the presence of glomerulus-like subregions in the LAL.[20] FLP-out labeling[54] applied to the ORN-specific *Or83b-Gal4* line[27,42] allowed to visualize individual ORNs in the background of the remaining, differently labeled ORNs.[15] Each ORN ended up invariably in a single LAL glomerulus, and FLP-out and background labels were always mutually exclusive (Fig. 2). This suggests that every glomerulus is the target of a single ORN and that each of the 21 ORNs is unique in projecting to its proper

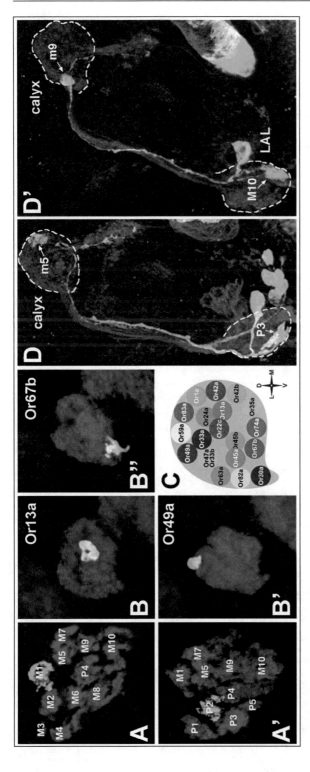

Figure 2. Dissection of the larval olfactory pathway by single cell analysis. (A,A') Terminals of two odorant receptor neurons (ORNs) in individual, annotated glomeruli of the LAL at the 3rd larval instar, visualized by FLP-out in the ORN-specific *Or83b-Gal4* line. ORNs that underwent FLP-mediated recombination are labeled in green; the remaining ORNs are labeled in magenta. Mutually exclusive green/magenta labeling demonstrates that each glomerulus is the target of a single ORN. (B,B',B'') In agreement with the FLP-out data, GFP reporter expression (green) driven by different *Or-Gal4* lines shows that each ORN targets a single, individual LAL glomerulus (3 examples shown). (C) Glomerular map of the LAL based on the terminals of different *Or-Gal4* lines. (D,D') Single projection neurons (PNs) labeled via FLP-out (in green) on top of other PNs (magenta). Essentially, each PN links a single glomerulus of the LAL with a single glomerulus of the mushroom body calyx. The two panels show that for many PNs, a given input glomerulus in the LAL (e.g., P3, M10) is correlated with a particular output glomerulus in the calyx (m5,m9). (A,A',D,D': reprinted from: Ramaekers A, Magnenat E, Marin EC et al. Glomerular maps without cellular redundancy at successive levels of the *Drosophila* larval olfactory circuit. Curr Biol 2005; 15:982-992. ©2006 with permission from Elsevier; B,B',B'',C: reprinted from: Fishilevich E, Domingos AI, Asahina K et al. Chemotaxis behavior mediated by single larval olfactory neurons in *Drosophila*. Curr Biol 2005; 15:2086-2096. ©2006 with permission from Elsevier.)

glomerulus among 21 spatially identifiable LAL glomeruli.[15] Compatible with the FLP-out data, the axons of ORNs expressing *Gal4* under the control of 22 different *Or* gene promoters ended up in a different glomerulus each (Fig. 2).[12,13] Moreover, combinations of two *Or-Gal4* driver constructs normally labeled two ORNs each of which projected to a different glomerulus. An obvious exception were *Or* genes coexpressed in the same ORN; these had a common glomerulus as a target. Having identified ligands for some of the ORs (see above), a map of odor representation in the LAL was established.[13] Accordingly, target glomeruli of receptors tuned to aliphatic compounds and target glomeruli of receptors tuned to aromatic compounds appeared to cluster at distinct sites of the LAL.

Using the same FLP-out strategy as for ORNs, but in the PN-specific GH146-*Gal4* driver,[55] the dendrites of larval PNs were found to be restricted to single LAL glomeruli, comparable to the adult antennal lobe (Fig. 2).[15] Using MARCM labeling,[56] a minority of PNs were found to be bi-glomerular.[52] Mutually exclusive FLP-out and background labels suggested that each glomerulus is innervated by a single GH146-positive PN. Hence, the total number of PNs may roughly match the total number of LAL glomeruli.[15] The glomeruli recognized by PNs correspond to those identified via the ORN terminals, indicating that LAL glomeruli meet the wiring criteria of typical insect glomeruli.

Glomerular Organization of the Mushroom Body Calyx

The adult MB calyx comprises hundreds of glomeruli.[57] Adult PNs establish 1-11 terminal boutons in variable calyx regions,[54] each bouton probably corresponding to a single glomerulus.[57] In contrast, the larval MB calyx consists of a small number of well-defined, relatively large glomeruli,[52] which has allowed to establish annotated glomerular maps. By expressing GFP-actin under the control of PN-specific and MB-specific *Gal4* lines or based on immunoreactivity patterns against choline acetyl transferase in the terminals of PNs, up to 34 calyx glomeruli were identified.[14,15] Fine structural data suggest that each calyx glomerulus is filled by a large, bouton-like terminal of a single PN.[52] Most of the PNs terminate in a single calyx glomerulus, except a minority of PNs which target two different glomeruli.[14,15,52] Again, calyx glomeruli seem to be innervated by single GH146-positive PNs.[15]

A comparison of the input and output sites of PNs revealed at least seven types of PNs that stereotypically link a specific LAL glomerulus with a specific calyx glomerulus (Fig. 2).[15] Thus, the activity pattern set up in LAL glomeruli, as a result of ORN input and modulation by local interneurons, seems to be rather faithfully transmitted to the calyx. This straightforward circuitry seems well suited for analyzing calyx function, although it remains to be shown whether strict input-output correlations apply to all larval PNs.

FLP-out and MARCM labeling in MB-specific *Gal4* lines allowed to classify MB γ neurons (the only type of mature MB neurons present in the larva[58]) according to their dendritic patterns in the calyx. While a minority of these neurons establish dendritic projections in a single calyx glomerulus,[15] most of them have multiple arbors in up to seven glomeruli.[14,15] When studying the MB γ neuron progenies deriving from the four MB neuroblasts, specific subsets of calyx glomeruli appeared to be preferentially targeted to some extent.[14] In terms of cell numbers, roughly 21 PNs (or perhaps a few more) may be confronted with an estimated 600 functional MB γ neurons (L. Luo, personal communication). Hence, the larval calyx, similar to its adult homologue, is a site of divergence;[14,15] it is in fact the only such site along the larval olfactory pathway (see Fig. 3).

The Larval Olfactory Pathway: Possible Rules of Odor Coding

As shown above, larval ORNs express only one or two *Or* genes along with the ubiquitously expressed *Or83b* gene.[12,13,27] This is similar to adult flies and mammals but differs from *C. elegans*, in which ORNs express multiple ORs.[59] By using "subtractive" and "additive" ORN strategies, possible rules of olfactory coding were investigated in larval chemotaxis assays.[12] In the first strategy, in which selected ORNs were genetically ablated via toxin expression, two types of results were obtained. Animals lacking the OR1a-expressing neuron or the OR49a-expressing neuron showed reduced chemotaxis to only one of 20 odors tested. This mild effect is consistent with the broad and overlapping ligand tuning of many ORNs in adults[39] and larvae.[13] In contrast, loss of the neuron expressing OR42a resulted in behavioral anosmy to four of the 20 odors. In the additive approach, larvae with one or two functional ORNs were generated using *Or1a*, *Or42a* or *Or49a* driver lines.[12] Consistent with the stronger OR42a-ablated phenotype, OR42a-functional larvae responded behaviorally to 22 of 53 odors tested (compared to 36 in the wildtype), including three of four odors to which OR42a-ablated animals are anosmic. The broad response profile for OR42a-functional larvae is in agreement with the broad ligand tuning of this receptor.[13,38] In contrast, OR1a- and OR49a-functional larvae did not exhibit significant chemotaxis to any of the 53 odors, consistent with the weak phenotype of the corresponding ablated larvae and with electrophysiological responses.[13] Animals with two functional ORNs (OR1a/OR42a) responded to a somewhat different subset of odors than larvae having either single functional neuron alone.[12]

The minimal effects on chemotaxis observed after ablating the OR1a or OR49a neurons suggest a certain degree of functional redundancy. This sounds surprising, given the small number of ORNs in the larval system. Yet, subtle effects exerted by seemingly "unimportant" neurons could be crucial for cooperative processes. On the other hand, the OR42a neuron plays a particularly important role; it is sufficient to initiate chemotaxis to many odors, and its loss leads to severe behavioral defects. Finally, cooperativity is suggested by the modified responses of OR1a/OR42a-functional animals compared to the single functional animals. Olfactory coding thus does not simply rely on additive activation of 21 parallel pathways, but involves lateral interactions as well. Cross-talk may occur in particular via the local interneurons in the LAL.[15] Transformation of olfactory signals is known from the antennal lobe of a number of insects including *Drosophila*.[60-63] Integration of olfactory information may sharpen quantitative and qualitative parameters, such as detection threshold and odor discrimination. While chemotaxis assays do not answer how odors are distinguished from each other, it is reasonable to assume that integrative processes may be particularly crucial if very few channels have to deal with many odors.

Further processing occurs in higher brain centers, such as the MBs. The different classes of larval MB γ neurons, innervating various numbers of calyx glomeruli, obviously allow different modes of signal transfer. Uniglomerular MB γ neurons may be involved in elementary coding of odor features, whereas multiglomerular MB γ neurons receiving input from several PNs may act as coincidence detectors.[14,15,64,65] Hence, although both LAL and larval calyx are glomerular, the logic of connectivity is different. LAL glomeruli exhibit stereotypic connectivity between defined ORNs and PNs, whereas calyx glomeruli show stereotypic input but mostly nonstereotypic, highly combinatorial MB γ neuron output.[14]

Distinctive Features of Larval and Adult Olfactory Circuits

Whereas the general design of the larval olfactory pathway is similar to its adult counterpart, larval ORNs and most (perhaps all) larval PNs appear to be unique, leading to an almost complete lack of cellular redundancy (Fig. 3). Consequently, any cell loss should affect olfactory function more severely than in the adult system. Moreover, the presence of no more than 21 ORNs and 21 LAL glomeruli suggests that the number of primary olfactory qualities in the larva is largely reduced compared to adults comprising about 50 glomeruli.[66] Also, given the uniglomerular projections of ORNs and PNs and the almost equal number of ORs, ORNs, LAL glomeruli, PNs and calyx glomeruli, the larval olfactory pathway lacks convergent and divergent connectivity up to the calyx and is organized in a 1:1:1:1:1 manner. This contrasts with the adult olfactory pathway, in which 1,300 ORNs converge onto about 50 glomeruli, which diverge again to approximately 150 PNs and hundreds of calyx glomeruli.[67,68] Convergence and cellular redundancy in sensory systems are known to increase the signal-to-noise ratio, whereas divergent connectivity very likely improves signal discrimination. In the larval olfactory system,

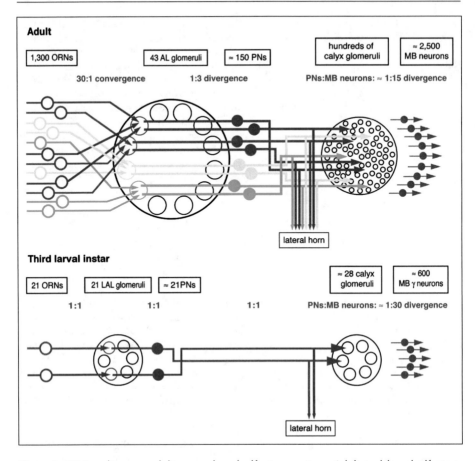

Figure 3. Wiring diagram: adult *versus* larval olfactory system. Adult and larval olfactory pathways are similarly organized. However, in the adult there are twice as many primary olfactory identities, represented by the types of odorant receptor neurons (ORNs, shown in different colors) or antennal lobe (AL) glomeruli. Moreover, in the adult, the different types of ORNs (open circles) and projection neurons (PNs; filled circles) that innervate a particular AL glomerulus exist as multiple copies, whereas larval ORNs and PNs are unique. Thus, the adult olfactory pathway is characterized by converging and diverging connectivity in the AL (ratios indicated refer to the features shown in the preceding line), while the larval pathway is organized as parallel channels without cellular redundancy. Hence, larval ORNs, LAL glomeruli, PNs and calyx glomeruli are related essentially in a 1:1:1:1 fashion. Reprinted from: Ramaekers A, Magnenat E, Marin EC et al. Curr Biol 2005; 15:982-992. ©2006 with permission from Elsevier[15].

the lack of cellular redundancy, the low number of input channels, and the absence of convergent/divergent LAL architecture are likely to reduce both the sensitivity and the signal-to-noise ratio. However, olfactory performance still seems sufficient for an animal that lives directly on its food substrate.

Gustatory System

Gustatory Receptors and Their Expression Pattern

In contrast to smell, taste deals with a very limited number of qualities, like "sweet" or "bitter". This characteristic is not due to a smaller diversity of existing tastants, but to the specific rationale of the gustatory system, which is designed for classifying substances rather than identifying particular molecules. This is particularly true for potentially harmful (bitter) compounds: they are chemically very diverse but should trigger the same behavioral response, i.e., aversion. It is therefore not surprising that in mammals receptor neurons tuned to such compounds express multiple types of gustatory receptors (GRs),[69] suggesting that the capacity of these cells to distinguish between different bitter substances is limited.

In adult *Drosophila*, evidence suggests that the GR family (see *Odorant Receptors and Their Expression Patterns*) mediates both sweet and bitter responses. Yet, because of low expression levels, *Gr* expression patterns were studied exclusively by *Gr* gene promoter-*Gal4* analysis.[35,36] Similar to mammals, neurons responding to sugars appear to express only one or a few GRs, whereas neurons that bind bitter compounds express multiple GRs.[70,71] This design allows to establish distinct attractive and aversive gustatory pathways. Surprisingly, three GRs are expressed on the antenna, suggesting that GRs are not strictly associated with taste function.[36] Indeed, the *Gr21a* gene is expressed in CO_2-sensitive cells of the antenna.[72]

From the few *Gr* genes that have been studied in the larva by promoter-*Gal4* analysis,[12,36] *Gr2a*, *Gr21a*, *Gr22e*, *Gr28be*, *Gr32a* and *Gr66a*—all of which are expressed also in the adult—show expression in one or two neurons of the TO (Table 1). *Gr2a* labels in addition two non-olfactory neurons of the DO. GR22e, GR28be, GR32a and GR66a were suspected to represent "bitter" receptors in the adult, as they are coexpressed in many neurons.[70,71] However, reporter expression driven by the gene promoter pairs *Gr66a/Gr21a* or *Gr66a/Gr32a* labeled two larval neurons each.[36] Yet, the small number of available data does not allow to draw any conclusion about the numbers of GRs expressed by individual neurons. Interestingly, the putative CO_2-receptor GR21a (see above), is expressed in the TO. Furthermore, *Gr2a* and several *Or* gene members (*Or30a, Or42a, Or49a, Or63a*), are expressed in both DO and TO.[12,13,36] Thus, as in adults, gene family membership and site of expression are not strictly linked. Finally, salt detection is mediated by degenerin/epithelial Na$^+$ channels, which are expressed in the TO as well as in adult taste bristles.[73]

Primary Gustatory Centers

Little is known about the organization of primary taste centers, mainly because they lack discrete glomerular architecture. In the adult, gustatory afferents from the pharynx, labellum and legs terminate in distinct regions of the suboesophageal ganglion (SOG).[70,71] Neurons from sensilla on different body regions projecting to different SOG regions may express the same GR, suggesting that the same tastant may trigger different behaviors, depending on the stimulation site. Labellar neurons expressing putative bitter receptors and labellar neurons expressing sugar receptors establish distinct but overlapping projections in the SOG.[70,71,74]

In the larva, the few existing data do not allow any meaningful generalizations. Yet, one TO neuron expressing *Gr32a* and three other neurons expressing *Gr66a*—one from the TO and two from pharyngeal sense organs—were shown to project to the ipsilateral SOG.[36] *Gr66a* and *Gr32a* projections are adjacent to each other but do not overlap. A third receptor, GR2a that is expressed in two DO neurons and one TO neuron, has two targets in the SOG.[36] This suggests again that a given tastant can elicit different behaviors depending on the stimulation site. It is also worth notifying that the *Gal4* lines *Or30a, Or42a,* and *Or49a* (Table 1) are not only expressed in the DO and TO, but also label sensory terminals in the SOG.[13]

Recently, a genetically defined subset of approximately 20 putative first-order gustatory target neurons was identified in the larval SOG.[75] These neurons provide output to the protocerebrum, the ventral nerve cord, the ring gland and pharyngeal muscles. They express the *hugin* gene, which generates two neuropeptides, and which appears to be upregulated in the absence of the feeding-regulatory transcription factor *klumpfuss* (P[9036]) and downregulated by amino acid-deficient conditions. Also, blocking the output from *hugin*-expressing neurons increases feeding. Apparently these neurons integrate taste processing, the endocrine system, higher-order brain centers and motor output. The dopaminergic nature of some of the *hugin*-expressing neurons[75] renders them interesting candidates as regulators of feeding, the most striking behavior of larvae.

The *Drosophila* Larva as a Model for Smell and Taste

The usefulness of *Drosophila* flies as an olfactory model system is obvious, given the genetic and molecular tools available, the simplicity of their olfactory system in terms of cell numbers and the striking similarities with the mammalian olfactory system. Surprisingly, even the larval olfactory system shares the design of the mammalian system, in the simplest conceivable form (Fig. 3). The larva may thus turn into a highly attractive "minimal" model for olfactory studies, in particular because it permits the generation of animals with a single functional ORN. In such larvae, odors, ORs, and ORNs can be directly correlated with behavioral output, allowing to track down the olfactory code to the level of identified receptor neurons.

The model character of *Drosophila* for the gustatory system is less obvious, both in adults and larvae. Anatomically, the taste systems of mammals and insects are different. Yet, there are a number of interesting parallels: (1) both insect and mammalian taste receptor neurons seem to be tuned to either attractive or aversive stimuli; (2) many more of the taste receptors may be dedicated to repulsive ligands than to attractive ones and, (3) cells responding to attractive cues seem to express only one or a few receptors, whereas those responding to bitter substances express multiple receptors.

The parallels in the chemosensory systems of vertebrates and insects are not necessarily evidence for a common ancestry. Rather, the similarities may reflect functional constraints for efficient smell and taste systems. Understanding these properties will surely aid understanding chemosensory function. In this context, *Drosophila* with its simple nervous system combined with a wealth of molecular tools, will contribute to our comprehension of smell and taste in general.

Acknowledgements

I am very grateful to N. Gendre (Fribourg) for providing Figure 1, and to B. Gerber (Würzburg) for comments on the manuscript. This work was supported by the Swiss National Fund (grants 31-63447.00, 3100A0-105517 and 3234-069273.02) and the Roche Research Foundation.

References

1. Buck L, Axel R. A novel multigene family may encode odorant receptors: a molecular basis for odor recognition. Cell 1991; 65:175-187.

2. Sengupta P, Chou JH, Bargmann CI. odr-10 encodes a seven transmembrane domain olfactory receptor required for responses to the odorant diacetyl. Cell 1996; 84:899-909.

3. Clyne PJ, Warr CG, Freeman MR et al. A novel family of divergent seven-transmembrane proteins: candidate odorant receptors in Drosophila. Neuron 1999; 22:327-338.

4. Vosshall LB, Amrein H, Morozov PS et al. A spatial map of olfactory receptor expression in the Drosophila antenna. Cell 1999; 96:725-736.

5. Ressler KJ, Sullivan SL, Buck LB. Information coding in the olfactory system: Evidence for a stereotyped and highly organized epitope map in the olfactory bulb. Cell 1994; 79:1245-1255.

6. Vassar R, Chao SK, Sitcheran R et al. Topographic organization of sensory projections to the olfactory bulb. Cell 1994; 79:981-991.

7. Gao Q, Yuan B, Chess A. Convergent projections of Drosophila olfactory neurons to specific glomeruli in the antennal lobe. Nat Neurosci 2000; 3:780-785.

8. Vosshall LB, Wong AM, Axel R. An olfactory sensory map in the fly brain. Cell 2000; 102:147-159.

9. Hildebrand JG, Shepherd G. Mechanisms of olfactory discrimination: converging evidence for common principles across phyla. Annu Rev Neurosci 1997; 20:595-631.

10. Strausfeld NJ, Hildebrand JG. Olfactory systems: common design, uncommon origins? Curr Opin Neurobiol 1999; 9:634-639.

11. Ache BW, Young JM. Olfaction: diverse species, conserved principles. Neuron 2005; 48:417-430.

12. Fishilevich E, Domingos AI, Asahina K et al. Chemotaxis behavior mediated by single larval olfactory neurons in Drosophila. Curr Biol 2005; 15:2086-2096.

13. Kreher SA, Kwon AY, Carlson JR. The molecular basis of odor coding in the Drosophila larva. Neuron 2005; 46:445-456.
14. Masuda-Nakagawa LM, Tanaka NK, O'Kane CJ. Stereotypic and random patterns of connectivity in the larval mushroom body calyx of Drosophila. Proc Natl Acad Sci USA 2005; 102:19027-19032.
15. Ramaekers A, Magnenat E, Marin EC et al. Glomerular maps without cellular redundancy at successive levels of the Drosophila larval olfactory circuit. Curr Biol 2005; 15:982-992.
16. Singh RN, Singh K. Fine structure of the sensory organs of Drosophila melanogaster Meigen Larva (Diptera: Drosophilidae). Int J Insect Morphol Embryol 1984; 13:255-273.
17. Schmidt-Ott U, Gonzalez-Gaitan M, Jäckle H et al. Number, identity, and sequence of the Drosophila head segments as revealed by neural elements and their deletion patterns in mutants. Proc Natl Acad Sci USA 1994; 91:8363-8367.
18. Campos-Ortega JA, Hartenstein V. The Embryonic Development of Drosophila melanogaster. Berlin, Heidelberg, New York: Springer, 1997.
19. Singh RN. Neurobiology of the gustatory systems of Drosophila and some terrestrial insects. Micr Res Techn 1997; 39:547-563.
20. Python F, Stocker RF. Adult-like complexity of the larval antennal lobe of D. melanogaster despite markedly low numbers of odorant receptor neurons. J Comp Neurol 2002; 445:374-387.
21. Gendre N, Lüer K, Friche S et al. Integration of complex larval chemosensory organs into the adult nervous system of Drosophila. Development 2004; 131:83-92.
22. Chu IW, Axtell RC. Fine structure of the dorsal organ of the house fly larva, Musca domestica L. Z Zellforsch Mikrosk Anat 1971; 117:17-34.
23. Chu-Wang IW, Axtell RC. Fine structure of the terminal organ of the house fly larva, Musca domestica L. Z. Zellforsch Mikrosk Anat 1972; 127:287-305.
24. Chu-Wang, IW, Axtell RC. Fine structure of the ventral organ of the house fly larva, Musca domestica L. Z Zellforsch Mikrosk Anat 1972; 130:489-495.
25. Oppliger FY, Guerin PM, Vlimant M. Neurophysiological and behavioural evidence for an olfactory function for the dorsal organ and a gustatory one for the terminal organ in Drosophila melanogaster larvae. J Insect Physiol 2000; 46:135-144.
26. Heimbeck G, Bugnon V, Gendre N et al. Smell and taste perception in D. melanogaster larva: toxin expression studies in chemosensory neurons. J Neurosci 1999; 19:6599-6609.
27. Larsson MC, Domingos AI, Jones WD et al. Or83b encodes a broadly expressed odorant receptor essential for Drosophila olfaction. Neuron 2004; 43:703-714.
28. Liu L, Yermolaieva O, Johnson WA et al. Identification and function of thermosensory neurons in Drosophila larvae. Nat Neurosci 2003; 6:267-273.
29. Kankel DR, Ferrus A, Garen SH et al. The structure and development of the nervous system. In: Ashburner M, Wright TRF, eds. The Genetics and Biology of Drosophila. London, New York, San Francisco: Academic Press, 1980:295-368.
30. Frederik RD, Denell RE. Embryological origin of the antenno-maxillary complex of the larva of Drosophila melanogaster Meigen. Int J Insect Morphol Embryol 1982; 11:227-233.
31. Tissot M, Gendre N, Hawken A et al. Larval chemosensory projections and invasion of adult afferents in the antennal lobe of Drosophila melanogaster. J Neurobiol 1997; 32:281-297.
32. Robertson HM, Warr CG, Carlson JR. Molecular evolution of the insect chemoreceptor gene superfamily in Drosophila melanogaster. Proc Natl Acad Sci USA 2003; 100:14537-14542.
33. Hallem EA, Dahanukar A, Carlson JR. Insect odor and taste receptors. Annu Rev Entomol 2006; 51:113-135.
34. Clyne PJ, Warr CG, Carlson JR. Candidate taste receptors in Drosophila. Science 2000; 287:1830-1834.
35. Dunipace L, Meister S, McNealy C et al. Spatially restricted expression of candidate taste receptors in the Drosophila gustatory system. Curr Biol 2001; 11:822-835.
36. Scott K, Brady R Jr, Cravchik A et al. A chemosensory gene family encoding candidate gustatory and olfactory receptors in Drosophila. Cell 2001; 104:661-673.
37. Dobritsa AA, van der Goes van Naters W, Warr CG et al. Integrating the molecular and cellular basis of odor coding in the Drosophila antenna. Neuron 2003; 37:827-841.
38. Goldman AL, van der Goes van Naters W, Lessing, D et al. Coexpression of two functional odor receptors in one neuron. Neuron 2005; 45:661-666.
39. Hallem EA, Ho MG, Carlson JR. The molecular basis of odor coding in the Drosophila antenna. Cell 2004; 117:965-979.
40. Bhalerao S, Sen A, Stocker RF et al. Olfactory neurons expressing identified receptor genes project to subsets of glomeruli within the antennal lobe of Drosophila melanogaster. J Neurobiol 2003; 54:577-592.

41. Fiala A, Spall T, Diegelmann S et al. Genetically expressed cameleon in Drosophila melanogaster is used to visualize olfactory information in projection neurons. Curr Biol 2002; 12:1877-1884.

42. Ng M, Roorda RD, Lima SQ et al. Transmission of olfactory information between three populations of neurons in the antennal lobe of the fly. Neuron 2002; 36:463-474.

43. Wang JW, Wong AM, Flores J et al. Two-photon calcium imaging reveals an odor-evoked map of activity in the fly brain. Cell 2003; 112:271-282.

44. Yu D, Ponomarev A, Davis RL. Altered representation of the spatial code for odors after olfactory classical conditioning: memory trace formation by synaptic recruitment. Neuron 2004; 42:437-449.

45. Couto A, Alenius M, Dickson BJ. Molecular, anatomical, and functional organization of the Drosophila olfactory system. Curr Biol 2005; 15:1535-1547.

46. Neuhaus E, Gisselmann G, Zhang W et al. Odorant receptor heterodimerization in the olfactory system of Drosophila melanogaster. Nat Neurosci 2004; 8:15-17.

47. Benton R, Sachse S, Michnick SW et al. Atypical membrane topology and heteromeric function of Drosophila odorant receptors in vivo. PLoS Biology 2005; 4(2):e20, DOI: 10.1371/journal pbio 004002046.

48. Komiyama T, Carlson JR, Luo L. Olfactory receptor neuron axon targeting: intrinsic transcriptional control and hierarchical interactions. Nat Neurosci 2004; 7:819-825.

49. Rodrigues V. Olfactory behavior of Drosophila melanogaster. In: Siddiqi O, Babu P, Hall LM, Hall JC, eds. Development and Neurobiology of Drosophila. New York, London: Plenum, 1980:361-371.

50. Monte P, Woodard C, Ayer R et al. Characterization of the larval olfactory response in Drosophila and its genetic basis. Behav Genet 1989; 19:267-283.

51. Cobb M. What and how do maggots smell? Biol Rev 1999; 74:425-459.

52. Marin EC, Watts RJ, Tanaka NK et al. Developmentally programmed remodeling of the Drosophila olfactory circuit. Development 2005; 132:725-737.

53. Python F, Stocker RF. Immunoreactivity against choline acetyltransferase, gamma-aminobutyric acid, histamine, octopamine, and serotonin in the larval chemosensory system of Drosophila melanogaster. J Comp Neurol 2002; 453:157-167.

54. Wong AM, Wang JW, Axel R. Spatial representation of the glomerular map in the Drosophila proto-cerebrum. Cell 2002; 109:229-241.

55. Stocker RF, Heimbeck G, Gendre N et al. Neuroblast ablation in Drosophila P[GAL4] lines reveals origins of olfactory interneurons. J Neurobiol 1997; 32:443-456.

56. Lee T, Luo L. Mosaic analysis with a repressible cell marker for studies of gene function in neuronal morphogenesis. Neuron 1999; 22:451-461.

57. Yasuyama K, Meinertzhagen IA, Schürmann FW. Synaptic organization of the mushroom body calyx in Drosophila melanogaster. J Comp Neurol 2002; 445:211-226.

58. Lee T, Lee A, Luo L. Development of the Drosophila mushroom bodies: sequential generation of three distinct types of neurons from a neuroblast. Development 1999; 126:4065-4076.

59. Troemel ER, Chou JH, Dwyer ND et al. Divergent seven transmembrane receptors are candidate chemosensory receptors in C. elegans. Cell 1995; 83:207-218.

60. Sachse S, Galizia CG. Role of inhibition for temporal and spatial odor representation in olfactory output neurons: a calcium imaging study. J Neurophysiol 2002; 87:1106-1117.

61. Lei H, Christensen TA, Hildebrand JG. Spatial and temporal organization of ensemble representations for different odor classes in the moth antennal lobe. J Neurosci 2004; 24:11108-11119.

62. Wilson RI, Turner GC, Laurent G. Transformation of olfactory representations in the Drosophila antennal lobe. Science 2004; 30:366-370.

63. Wilson RI, Laurent G. Role of GABAergic inhibition in shaping odor-evoked spatiotemporal patterns in the Drosophila antennal lobe. J Neurosci 2005; 25:9069-9079.

64. Perez-Orive J, Mazor O, Turner GC et al. Oscillations and sparsening of odor representations in the mushroom body. Science 2002; 297:359-365.

65. Heisenberg M. Mushroom body memoir: from maps to models. Nat Revs Neurosci 2003; 4:266-275.

66. Laissue PP, Reiter C, Hiesinger PR et al. Three-dimensional reconstruction of the antennal lobe in Drosophila melanogaster. J Comp Neurol 1999; 405:543-552.

67. Stocker RF. The organization of the chemosensory system in Drosophila melanogaster: a review. Cell Tiss Res 1994; 275:3-26.

68. Stocker RF. Drosophila as a focus in olfactory research: mapping of olfactory sensilla by fine structure, odor specificity, odorant receptor expression and central connectivity. Micr Res Techn 2001; 55:284-296.

69. Montmayeur JP, Matsunami H. Receptors for bitter and sweet taste. Curr Opin Neurobiol 2002; 12:366-371.

70. Thorne N, Chromey C, Bray S et al. Taste perception and coding in Drosophila. Curr Biol 2004; 14:1065-1079.

71. Wang Z, Singhvi A, Kong P et al. Taste representations in the Drosophila brain. Cell 2004; 117:981-991.
72. Suh GSB, Wong AM, Hergarden AC et al. A single population of olfactory sensory neurons mediates an innate avoidance behavior in Drosophila. Nature 2004; 431:854-859.
73. Liu L, Leonard AS, Motto DG et al. Contribution of Drosophila DEG/ENaC genes to salt taste. Neuron 2003; 39:133-146.
74. Marella S, Fischler W, Kong P et al. Imaging taste responses in the fly brain reveals a functional map of taste category and behavior. Neuron 2006; 49:285-295.
75. Melcher C, Pankratz MJ. Candidate gustatory interneurons modulating feeding behavior in the Drosophila brain. PLoS Biol 2005; 3(9):e305, DOI: 10.1371/journal pbio 0030305.

CHAPTER 6

Development of the *Drosophila* Olfactory System

Veronica Rodrigues and Thomas Hummel*

Abstract

The olfactory system throughout the animal kingdom is characterized by a large number of highly specialized neuronal cell types. Olfactory receptor neurons (ORNs) in the peripheral sensory epithelium display two main differentiation features: the selective expression of a single odorant receptor out of a large genomic repertoire of receptor genes and the synaptic connection to a single type of relay neuron in the primary olfactory CNS target area. In the mouse olfactory system, odorant receptors themselves play a central role in the coordination of both types of ORN differentiation. The olfactory system of *Drosophila*, although similar in structural and functional organization compared to mammals, does not seem to involve odorant receptors in the selection of OR gene expression and target cell recognition, suggesting distinct developmental control mechanisms. In this chapter we summarize recent findings in *Drosophila* of how gene networks regulate ORN specification and differentiation in the peripheral sensory organs as well as how different cellular interactions and patterning signals organize the class-specific axonal and dendritic connectivity in the CNS target area.

Introduction

An essential function of the nervous system is to receive vital information about the environment through different sensory channels. To create a faithful internal representation of the external world in the brain, the highly selective incoming information must be organized in a meaningful manner, which requires that presynaptic inputs be matched to appropriate postsynaptic outputs.[1] A well-studied example of neuronal sensory and synaptic specificity is the olfactory system. Molecular cloning of olfactory receptors (ORs) in vertebrates has provided valuable insights into the functional and anatomical organization of the olfactory system,[2] including the projection of olfactory receptor neurons (ORNs) from the olfactory epithelium to the primary synaptic target in the CNS, the olfactory bulb (OB). In mice, the olfactory epithelium contains about a 1000 different classes of ORNs defined by a unique OR expression.[3-5] ORNs of a given sensory specificity intermingle with those of different OR classes in the olfactory epithelium, but send their axons to a distinct primary synaptic target unit in the olfactory bulb brain region.[6,7] Although it is now well established that in mice ORs function in ORN axon-axon segregation in a local, contextual fashion,[6,8,9] the mechanism underlying terminal axon sorting remains obscure. The results of two recent studies have integrated the role of ORs and classical neuronal adhesion molecules in explaining how discrete identities of ORNs are converted into a spatial map of axonal connections.[10,11]

The adult olfactory system of *Drosophila* displays the same degree of sensory and synaptic specificity compared to vertebrates (Fig. 1), but with a reduced numerical complexity making it

*Corresponding Author: Thomas Hummel—Institut fuer Neurobiologie, Universitaet Muenster, Badestrasse 9, D-48149 Muenster, Germany. Email: hummel@uni-muenster.de

Brain Development in Drosophila melanogaster, edited by Gerhard M. Technau.
©2008 Landes Bioscience and Springer Science+Business Media.

an excellent experimental model to determine developmental control mechanisms.[12-19] The recent flurry of research on *Drosophila* olfactory system development and function has been catalyzed by the discovery and analysis of odorant receptor genes by the laboratories of Leslie Vosshall, John Carlson and Andrew Chess (reviewed in Laissue and Vosshall, this issue and references there-in).

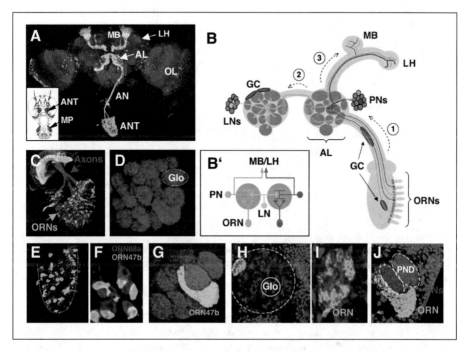

Figure 1. Organization of the *Drosophila* adult olfactory system. A) Whole mount preparation of the developing adult *Drosophila* brain, showing the projections of olfactory receptor neurons (ORNs) from the antenna (ANT) through the antennal nerve (AN) into the antennal lobe (AL), which is localized just ventrally to the mushroom body (MB) neuropil. The position of the lateral horn (LH) and the optic lobe (OL) is indicated. The inset indicates the position of the two olfactory appendages, the antenna (ANT) and the maxillary palp (MP). (B, B') Schematic drawing of the neuronal circuitry in the olfactory system: 1) Antennal ORN project their axons, associated with different types of glial cells (GCs), into the ipsi-lateral AL and axons converge into glomeruli according to the OR expression (red and green ORN class). B') Inside each glomerulus, ORN axon terminal branches interact with dendrites of Projection Neurons (PNs, mostly uni-glomerular projections) and Local Interneurons (LNs, multi-glomerular projections). 2) Most ORN classes send a projection across the commissure to innervate the corresponding glomerulus in the contra-lateral AL. 3) PNs transmit the olfactory information along their axons onto the MBs and neurons of the LH. Glial cells (GCs) cover the surface of the AL and send processes into the synaptic AL. C) Organization of ORN projections into three main fascicles in the third antennal segment. D) Subdivision of the AL neuropil into glomerular synaptic units (Glo), which can be individually recognized based on their position, size and shape. E) Distribution of two ORN classes (47b and 88a) across the antennal surface. ORN47b and ORN88a are localized together in the same sensillum (F) and project to neighboring glomeruli in the AL (G). H, I) Multi-glomerular innervation of LN dendrites (red) in the AL (dotted line). ORN axon terminals (green) occupy a region inside the glomerulus different from LN dendritic branches (red). J) A group of three glomeruli is shown, occupied by two classes of PNs (red, dotted lines) and a non-overlapping innervation by an ORN class (green). Red labeling: N-Cadherin (A,D), CD2 (E-J), 22C10 (C); Green labeling: GFP (A-J).

The G-coupled ORs are encoded by a family of ~60 genes each of which is expressed in a subset of ORNs.[20,21] Unlike the mammalian ORNs, where OR choice is believed to be stochastic,[22] expression in *Drosophila* neurons is defined by a combinatorial code of transcription factors some of which also play a role in determination of sense organ-type.[23] It therefore becomes necessary to understand how gene networks act to specify sense organs and determine cell fate in the olfactory system; this will be discussed in the first part of this review. Further, we now know that targeting of the ORNs is 'receptor-topic' where neurons expressing a given receptor wire to the same glomerulus(i) in the antennal lobe thus forming the basis of odor encoding (reviewed in ref. 17). The mechanisms that control this projection pattern and the development of the olfactory circuits are the subject of the second part of this review. For a more comprehensive view on olfactory system morphological and functional organization in the adult *Drosophila* see accompanied chapter by Laissue and Vosshall. The characteristics of the *Drosophila* larval olfactory system are discussed in the chapter by R. Stocker.

Organization of the *Drosophila* Adult Olfactory System

In adult *Drosophila melanogaster*, two types of, bilaterally symmetric, peripheral sensory appendages, the antenna and maxillary palpus, carry about 1200 and 120 ORNs respectively (Figs. 1A,2A).[13,14] The ORNs send their axons, associated with different types of peripheral glial cells (GCs), via the antennal and labial nerve towards the antennal lobe (AL; Fig. 1A-C). Here, all axons of a single ORN class that express the same OR send terminal synaptic branches into one out of about 50 glomeruli,[16,24-26] individually recognizable by a characteristic size, shape and position inside the AL (Fig. 1D,G).[27] Axons of most ORN classes show, in addition to the ipsi-lateral innervation, an extension across the dorsal commissure to contact the identical glomerulus in the contra-lateral AL (Fig. 1B).[28] Beside the terminal branches of ORN axons, each of the 50 glomerular units in the adult antennal lobe contains the processes of three additional cell types: the dendritic arborizations of Projections Neurons (PNs) and Local Interneurons (LNs) as well as different glial cells (GCs), which insulate individual glomeruli and also send processes into the glomerulus compartment[28-31] (Fig. 1B,B′). The cholinergic PNs are the main relay neurons in the AL, which transduce olfactory information to the Mushroom Bodies (MBs) and the Lateral Horn (LH). While most of the roughly 200 PNs display uni-glomerular dendritic projections (Fig. 1J), a group of multi-glomerular PNs in the ventral cluster has been described.[32,33] In contrast, multi-glomerular dendritic innervation is the main feature of the LNs to modulate the transmission of olfactory information between ORNs and PNs (Fig. 1B′,H,I). Although the organization of LNs in the adult AL is less well characterized compared to PNs, distinct morphological and functional (e.g., excitatory and inhibitory) classes have been identified.[34-37] Studies in other insects have shown that these different axonal and dendritic elements establish a complex synaptic network in which almost any connectivity permutation is possible (Fig. 1B′).[38-40]

Specification of the Olfactory Sense Organs

Olfactory sense organs are sensilla bearing 4-20 μm cuticular protuberances with microscopic pores or grooves presumably allowing entry of odorants into the sensillar lymph.[41] There are ~450 sensilla (~419 in males and ~457 in females), located on the third segment of the antenna with ~60 on the maxillary palp.[13,42] These are of three main morphological types—the trichoidea, basiconica, coleoconica—and a less well-defined intermediate type (Fig. 2A-D). Sensilla basiconica are innervated by either two or four neurons, coeloconica by two or three and trichoidea by between one and three neurons. Electrophysiological responses from single sense organs have classified ORNs into functional types based on their response to chemical components of food and pheromones as well as CO_2 and humidity.[43-48] The neuronal composition and properties of a sense organ at a particular position on the antennal surface is conserved between different animals suggesting a link between mechanisms that determine sense organ specification and positional cues that form the antenna.

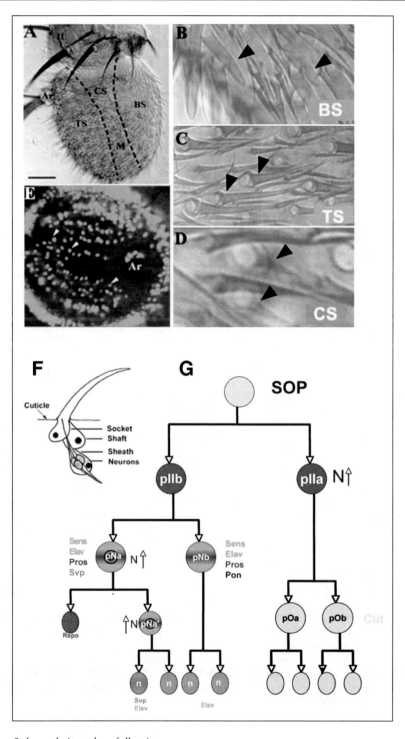

Figure 2, legend viewed on following page.

Figure 2, viewed on previous page. Organization and development of *Drosophila* olfactory sensilla. (A-D) Cuticular mounts of the third segment of the antenna showing the location of Basiconic sensilla (BS), Coeloconic sensilla (CS) and Trichoid sensilla (TS). Appropriate regions are enlarged in (B-D) to show the morphology of these sensilla (arrowheads). The regions demarcated in (A) are enriched in specific sensilla while all kinds are found in the mixed region (M). Large mechanosensory bristles are found on the second segment (II) and the arista (Ar) is believed to be involved in humidity and sound detection. E) Antennal disc at 8 hours APF (After Pupae Formation) from a *neuA101* animal stained with antibodies against β-galactosidase. The location of sensory progenitors is detected. F) Schematic diagram of a single sense organ. The sense organ is composed of a socket and shaft cell and is innervated by up to four neurons. Processes of the sheath cell wrap around the neuronal cell bodies at the base of the sensillum. G) Lineage of a single olfactory sense organ based on data from Endo et al (2006) and Sen et al (2003). The glial cell originates in all lineages but survives only when it originates in the coeloconic lineage. Neuron number is regulated by programmed cell death and can range between one and four neurons.

The adult antenna and maxillary palp develop from the eye-antennal disc; antennal identity is specified by the combinatorial action of the homeodomain proteins Homothorax, Extradenticle and Distalless and the basic helix-loop-helix (bHLH) protein Spineless (reviewed in ref. 49). The co-ordinates of the disc are established through the action of a hierarchy of patterning genes notably *engrailed, wingless, decapentaplegic* and *hedgehog* (reviewed in ref. 50). The interplay of these genes with the epidermal growth factor (EGF) signaling pathway leads to setting up a prepattern upon which the proneural genes act to select sense organ progenitors[51] (reviewed in refs. 52,53).

Olfactory progenitors are specified by two transcription factors—Atonal (Ato) and Amos—which possess bHLH domains for dimerization and DNA binding.[54,55] Null alleles of *ato* lack coeloconica, while mutations in *amos* affect the trichoid and basiconic sensilla on the antenna; the olfactory sensilla on the maxillary palp are specified by *ato*. The selection of a single sensory progenitor from an undifferentiated field of epidermal cells in the antennal disc shares similarities with mechanisms used in other well described sense organs in the peripheral nervous system.[56] The spatial expression of Ato and Amos in proneural domains is regulated by early genes that pattern the disc epidermis,[51] as well as negative regulators like Extramacrochaete.[55] Ato and Amos function require the activity of an additional bHLH protein Daughterless and the proneural domain is refined to single cell through Notch signaling.[54,55,57]

The formation of sense organs within the disc epidermis has been studied by following reporter expression in the *neuralised*[A101] (*neu*[A101]) line, which labels progenitor cells and their progeny (Fig. 2E)[58] and the expression of Senseless, which is a faithful indicator of proneural function.[59] Progenitors are specified in three temporal waves within the antennal disc first appearing a few hours before formation of the pupa. Early appearing progenitors are specified by *ato* and mutations result in an absence of these progenitors combined with defects in fascicle formation of the remaining ORNs.[30] Amos expression is detected in progenitors that arise in the third wave of sensillogenesis. In strong *amos* mutants sensilla trichoidea and basiconica are absent and the surface bears ectopic mechanosensory bristles.[59] Achaete (Ac) and Scute (Sc), which specifies the sense organ progenitors of mechanosensory bristles, becomes ectopically expressed in mutant discs suggesting that Amos acts to suppress *ac/sc* in the antenna.

The Runt family transcription factor Lozenge (Lz) activates the expression of *amos*.[54] Double mutants of *amos* and *lz* do not form ectopic mechanosensory bristles suggesting that Lz participates in the regulation of *ac/sc* expression.[59] Loss-of-function and gain-of-function analysis led to the model that specification of sensilla basiconica requires high levels of Lz while lower levels form sensilla trichoidea.[60] Lz has recently been shown to be an important regulator of Or gene expression in subsets of ORNs, thus providing a link between mechanisms that determine sense organ specificity and receptor gene selection.[23]

Olfactory Lineages Revisited

A typical olfactory sense organ is composed of three support cells—shaft (trichogen), socket (tormogen) and sheath (thecogen)—and is innervated by up to four neurons (Fig. 2F). Serial reconstruction of sections through a single sensillum often revealed the presence of an additional support cell, which probably is a second sheath cell.[61] The lineage of the cells within the olfactory sensillum has been difficult to decipher since a large number of sense organs develop asynchronously within the relatively small area of the antennal disc. Most of the early studies had examined the lineage of the olfactory sensilla by marking sensory cells using cellular reporters and antibodies.[58,62] β-galactosidase expression in the *neu*[A101] enhancer-trap line marks isolated progenitor cells, which are recognizable by their large apically placed nuclei.[58] The numbers of these cells increased into early pupation suggesting continual specification of precursors. 5-bromodeoxyuridine when injected into the haemolymph of animals aged between 0 and 12 hours after pupa formation (APF) was not incorporated into the sensory cells. On the other hand, this method as well as observation of dividing chromosomes with DAPI and phosphorylated histone immunocytochemistry provided evidence for a high level of proliferation among the dividing sensory cells at 14 and 16 hours APF. A model to explain these results suggested that sensory organ progenitors (also termed founder cells) did not divide but that a cluster of three or four cells (termed the presensillum cluster) divided to form the cells composing a single sense organ.[57,58,63] These conclusions are subject to errors since it was not possible to follow cells within a single cluster within a crowded epidermal field.

This difficulty has been solved recently by Endo and his colleagues[64] by exploiting the MARCM method[65,66] to mark progenitors and follow them during development. Heat-shock induction of Flipase activity at about 30 hours before pupation generated clones in all cells of a sense organ suggesting that these cells arise from a single progenitor cell (Fig. 2G). Examination of four-cell clones revealed two apical cells recognized by the external cell marker Cut and two basal cells, which express Senseless (Sens). The external, Cut positive cells denoted pOa and pOb arise by division of the secondary progenitor pIIa, while the Sens positive pNa and pNb arise from pIIb.

Sen et al[63] described clusters of 3 cells in the ~12 hour APF antenna labeled with *neu*[A101] of which two expressed the neuronal marker Elav and Prospero (Pros). This can be explained in the light of the findings of Endo et al,[64] by proposing that the secondary progenitors, like those in the mechanosensory lineages on the *Drosophila* notum, divide out of sync.[67,68] When three-cell clones were observed by Endo and his colleagues (personal communication), these consisted of a large cell (~4.0 μm in diameter) labeled weakly by anti-Sens and two smaller cells (~3.5 μm in diameter) both strongly labeled with anti-Sens, only one of which expressed partner of Numb (Pon). The large cell is possibly pIIa while the smaller cells are likely to be the progeny of pIIb—pNa and pNb—both of which express Elav and Pros. One of the two Pros expressing cells, which we denote as pNa, also expresses the orphan receptor Seven-up (Svp). Asymmetric segregation of Pros was observed in some clusters and a daughter cell inherited Svp and Pros transiently before staining with antibodies against the glial marker Reverse Polarity (Repo).[63]

This leads us to propose that pNa divides prior to pNb to form a glial cell and an additional progenitor pNa' which in turns divides to form two neurons, one of which continues to express Svp. This additional division has been proposed to explain observations by Sen et al (2003) that a cell that expresses Pros/Elav/Svp divides to form another cell that expresses these markers and a sibling that expresses Repo (Fig. 2G). The model explains the formation of four neurons which is the maximum number innervating a single olfactory sense organ. In sensory clusters with a small number of neurons (one, two or three) additional cells are presumably removed by programmed cell death which has been observed at time points corresponding to the differentiation of olfactory neurons.[57]

The distinction between the neuronal (pIIb) and nonneuronal (pIIa) lineages is determined by Notch signaling. Notch loss-of-function, generated either by mutations in the downstream activator *mastermind*,[64] a hypomorphic allele of *Notch-N*[ts] or ectopic expression of Numb[63] resulted in a pIIa to pIIb conversion leading to additional neural cells at the expense of external cells. In *nb* mutant clones two neurons expressing Svp were observed indicating a conversion of

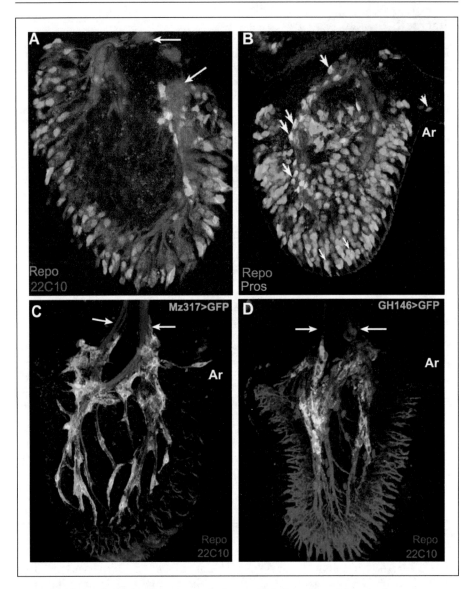

Figure 3. Glial cells in the antenna. At 36 hours APF, the sense organs in the antenna appear fully differentiated and ORNs can be identified by mAb22C10 staining (A,C,D). Axon bundles transit the third segment in distinct fascicles (long arrows). Prospero is expressed in two nonneuronal cells in each sensory cluster (blue in B). Glial cells stained with antibodies against Repo line the axonal bundles in the third segment (A; small arrows in B). The glial cells are of two subtypes: those labeled with *Mz317-Gal4* (C) and the *GH146-Gal4* subset (D). Ar-Arista.

pNb to pNa.[64] This implies that neuronal cells generated from pNa experience high N signaling while those from pNb are low in N levels. This binary switch in N signaling levels could act in differentiation of two populations of neurons within a single sensillum. This has importance in regulation of the wiring of ORNs to their glomerular targets and will be discussed later.[64] The role of Pros in pNa and pNb is unclear although its absence in the pIIa lineage is expected since Tramtrack, one of the targets of N signaling is known to suppress Pros expression.[69,70] Ectopic expression of Pros in all progenitors leads to an absence of external sensory structures suggesting defects in the pIIa lineage of cells. In differentiated sense organs, Pros expresses in nuclei of two of the support cells and loss-of-function clones produce twinned sensory shafts and sockets.[63] Svp expression is detected in pNa and mis-expression also affects the formation of the external sensory structures. Expression persists in one neuron in most sensory clusters, the function of which is not known (Fig. 2G).

Origin of Glial Cells

At 36 hours APF, the antenna appears to be fully differentiated and shows the presence of ORNs, which exit the antenna towards the brain in three distinct fascicles (Fig. 1C, 3A). There are ~100 glial cells that lie along the ORNs as they exit the antenna (Fig. 3B-D). In situations where N signaling is reduced during pupal development, the number of glial cells within the antenna was greatly increased. Since Repo+cells originate after division of a Pros/Elav/Svp expressing progenitor, we propose that these originate from the pNa cell shown in Fig. 2G. This additional division in the gliogenic lineage is reminiscent of the described division patterns in the mechanosensory lineages on the adult notum.[68,71]

In the adult antenna, total loss of *ato* function leads to an absence of coeloconic sensilla and a concomitant reduction in about 70 of the 100 glial cells. These glial presumably arise from the lineages specified by *ato* and influence the fasciculation of the olfactory receptor neurons.[72] The other lineages specified by the proneural gene Amos also produce glial cells but these undergo apoptosis soon after birth.[63] The Ato-dependent glial cells are labeled by the *Mz317-Gal4>GFP* stock (Fig. 3C). *GH146-Gal4* labels an independent subset of glia (Fig. 3D); indirect evidence suggests that these glial cells arise outside the antenna and migrate into the third antennal segment later in development.[73] The function of these cells is not yet known (see below).

Development of ORN Connectivity

The ORN axons projecting along the antennal nerve reach the developing AL at about 18-20 h after pupae formation (APF).[31] At the ventro-lateral AL entry point (Fig. 4A), ORN axons sort

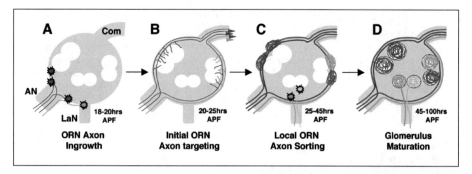

Figure 4. Development of ORN connectivity in the AL. A) Antennal ORN axons first reach the AL at about 18 hours APF and sort into a lateral and a medial pathway at the antennal nerve (AN) exit point. B) ORN axons bypass their prospective target area (white circles) as they project towards and across the dorsal commissure (com), but extend spatially restricted colateral processes. C) At about 30-35 hours APF, the first maxillary ORN axons reach the AL through the labial nerve (LaN), while the antennal ORN axons start to converge into protoglomeruli and shortly afterwards fuse with the dendritic field. D) In the second half of pupal development (45-100 hours APF), ORNs establish synaptic contacts and glial processes isolate individual glomeruli.

out, turn either into a medial or a lateral direction and continue to project in two broad pathways across the surface of the AL towards the dorso-medial corner,[29] (TH, unpublished observation). Inside these axon tracks, ORN axons initially bypass their prospective glomerular target area to project across the dorsal commissure, but individual axons extend small collateral processes in the region of their class-specific convergence (Fig. 4B).[74] The first axons cross the midline and extend into the contra-lateral AL by about 20 hours APF. ORN axons stay within the peripheral nerve fiber layer over the next 15 hours (Fig. 4C). During this period, the collateral axonal extension elongate followed by a sequential, spatially restricted process of axon condensation into increasingly discrete protoglomeruli that spreads across the developing AL.[74] These axonal protoglomeruli then begin to merge with the dendritic field of projection neurons so that by around 35 hours the first glomeruli can be distinguished and by 50 hours APF most glomeruli have formed (Fig. 4D).[31,74] Compared to the antenna, ORNs from the maxillary palps develop later and maxillary axons reaching the AL around 30 h APF at a ventral position to integrate into the antennal glomerular field (Fig. 4C).[75] Following the assembly of ORN axons and PN dendrites into glomeruli during the first half of pupal development, glomerulus maturation occurs in the remaining two days of the pupal phase, in which OR genes are turned on in the antenna and ORN axons form synapses in the antennal lobe (Fig. 4D).[76,77]

Olfactory Map Organization

The highly specific *Drosophila* olfactory circuit, composed of 50 individual channels, each of which is organized by the convergence of about 30 ORN axons, presents a fascinating wiring problem. Although the ORN projections from the periphery onto the glomerular array follow the principle of a discrete sensory map,[78] in which axons from spatially dispersed neurons with the same sensory identity project onto one location in the target field, some more global organization domains have been noticed.

As the different sensilla classes occupy distinct areas on the antenna, with the basiconic sensilla broadly located along the medial antennal surface and the trichoids more restricted to the lateral antennal areas (Fig. 2A), the topography of ORNs in the peripheral epithelium is approximately maintained in their projection into the brain (Fig. 5).[25] Although ORN axons do not fasciculate in the antenna strictly according to sensillum type, the 3 main fascicles described above contain ORN axons from the sensillum type enriched regions on the antennal surface (Fig. 5A, TH unpublished). When ORN axons reach the brain they defasciculate and become reorganized into several axon pathways with different medio-lateral positions across the AL surface: basiconic ORNs accumulate in the medial tracts and trichoid ORNs in the lateral tracts (Fig. 5B).[25] In *Manduca*, a special class of glial cells, important for ORN axon projection, has been identified that are located where the antennal nerve enters the AL.[79,80] It is tempting to speculate that, in *Drosophila*, the GH146-positive glial cells described above, are involved in this reorganization of ORN axon projection.[73]

Inside these sensilla-specific AL domains, the spatial organization of ORN classes in the periphery is not maintained and ORN classes which are housed in the same sensillum often project to glomeruli which are localized quite some distance apart.[25,26] Nevertheless, the ORN class specific axon convergence in the AL seem to be linked to cell fate specification in the course of differential divisions by the SOP progeny. The diversification of ORN precursors in the SOP lineage through the differential activation of the Notch signalling pathway (see above) does not only lead to a differential OR expression but also correlate with the global organization of ORN axon projection.[64] Endo and collaborators showed that axonal projections of "high-Notch" and "low-Notch" ORN classes segregate into a few multi-glomerular domains along the dorso-ventral AL axis (Fig. 5C). The subdivision of ORN class connectivity into different global domains along the dorso-ventral and medial-lateral axis suggest that a series of hierarchical decisions are made by ORN axons on their way from the peripheral sensory epithelium to the synaptic target region (see below). These sequentially acting signalling mechanisms would reduce the complexity to generate ORN synaptic specificity, leading to the positioning of ORN axons into a selected AL area, where local cues organizes the ORN class specific convergence.

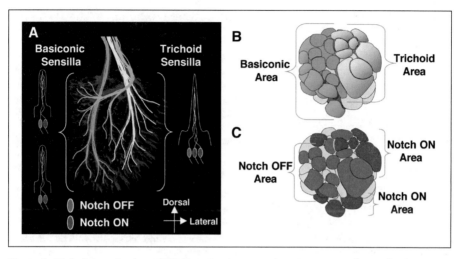

Figure 5. Global organization of ORN projections into the AL. A) ORNs housed in basiconic sensilla are enriched on the medial antennal surface and project into two main fascicles (blue and green) towards the AL. Trichoid sensilla neuronal projections from the lateral antennal surface are enriched in the third main fascicle (yellow). The ORNs of each sensillum can be subdivided into one "Notch OFF" neuron and one to three "Notch ON" neurons based on the position within the SOP lineage (see text). The axonal projections of "Notch OFF"- and "Notch ON"-type ORNs are intermingled within each of the three fascicles. B) The overall topographic organization of basiconic and trichoid ORNs is maintained in the ORN axon projections in the AL. C) "Notch OFF"- and "Notch ON"-type ORNs segregate into broad glomerular domains along the dorso-ventral axis. Red staining in A: 22C10-positive ORNs.

Cellular and Molecular Mechanisms of ORN Wiring Specificity

Recent progress in understanding the molecular basis of ORN wiring specificity has been achieved through the systematic use of an inducible genetic mosaic system (MARCM),[65,66] in which gene functions can be specifically removed from projecting ORNs (Fig. 5A-C). The induction of MARCM clones under the control of the *eyeless* promotor generates large regions of homozygous ORNs in the antennal epithelium but does not affect the precursors of the PNs and LNs in the developing AL.[81] In addition, the expression of Flipase under heat-shock (*hs*) promotor control enables the generation of single homozygous ORNs as well the induction of genetic mosaics in different populations of AL neurons.[82] This mosaic system has been used to address many aspects of olfactory system development, e.g., the origin of the different cell types and their clonal relationship in the antenna and AL,[64,83] the functional interplay of axons and dendrites during axonal and dendritic wiring[82,84,85] and the characterization of candidate genes in this cell-cell communication process.[86] Axonal connectivity phenotypes of candidate molecules (see below) and a large-scale histological screen (TH unpublished) further support the idea that hierarchical mechanisms control ORN axon targeting in the AL. Most mutant phenotypes can be classified as global or local misprojection (Fig. 6 D-I), suggesting that there are distinct and sequentially acting signalling mechanisms in which initial axon guidance to a coarse region of the AL is followed by local interactions that control the final refinement and precise matching of pre-and postsynaptic neuronal processes.

The first neuronal guidance molecules that have been shown to be required within ORNs are Dscam, a member of the Ig-domain superfamily and two Dscam downstream effectors, the SH2/SH3 adapter Dock and the serine/threonine kinase Pak.[81,87] All three genes are broadly expressed in the developing peripheral and central olfactory system. In *eyFlp* mosaics, *Dscam* mutant ORN axons still follow an approximately normal path across the antennal lobe, but converge prematurely at ectopic locations. Interestingly, they do not integrate into existing glomeruli at these ectopic sites; rather multiple *Dscam* mutant ORN axons converge to form novel glomerulus-like structures.[81] Labeling of multiple ORN classes revealed that *Dscam* mutant ORN axons segregate at ectopic sites, even outside the AL, in an ORN class specific manner (Fig. 6F-G ') indicating the existence of a unique axonal identity independent of the target area, which is counteracted by the Dscam activity (Fig. 6J; T.H. unpublished observations). *dock* and *Pak* mutant ORN axons show a more severe phenotype in which they grow along inappropriate pathways and therefore form ectopic terminations all over the AL. The Robo receptors are a second class of guidance molecules involved in the initial coarse targeting of ORN axons. Robo, Robo2 and Robo3 are expressed in discrete subsets of ORN axons that segregate from one another and take different medial versus lateral pathways across the developing AL.[29] Widespread mistargeting defects when Robo receptors are removed from ORNs or ectopically expressed suggest a crucial role for Robo signalling in ORN axon positioning.

Following the crude and overlapping positioning of ORN axon terminals of different classes within a restricted AL domain, local short-range *inter* and *intra*-class interactions lead to the class—specific axon sorting into protoglomeruli (Fig. 4C). Compared to the mutations described above, removal of the transmembrane molecule Semaphorin-1a and the Ca-dependent cell adhesion molecule N-Cadherin leads to more local axon targeting defects (Fig. 6H-I '). *Ncad* mutant ORN axons reach the vicinity of their AL target area, but the initial axonal convergence into protoglomeruli is disrupted; this in turn affects all subsequent steps of glomerulus maturation and axon-dendrite interaction finally results in a severe disorganisation of the adult AL neuropil.[74] However, N-Cadherin does not appear to mediate class-specific interactions between different ORN axons; rather it seems to be a permissive factor for axonal interactions among all ORNs.[74] In contrast to N-Cadherin, *Sema-1a* mutant ORN axons are able to induce local convergence, but axons of the same class split into multiple adjacent glomeruli or coconverge with ORN axons of neighboring glomeruli (Fig. 6H-I ').[75,88] Whereas N-Cadherin is ubiquitously expressed on projecting ORN axons, ORN axons converging into neighbouring glomeruli display different levels of Semaphorin-1a.[88] Clonal analysis indicates a non-autonomous Sema-1a function, mediated through the Plexin A receptor, onto neighbouring classes, most likely in a repulsive fashion. In summary, different types of inter-axonal attractive (via N-Cadherin) and repulsive (via Dscam and Sema-1a/Plexin A) interactions, lead to a final coalescence of ORN axons in OR type specific protoglomeruli (Fig. 6J).

Specification of Projection Neurons

In contrast to ORN formation during pupal development, the generation of the olfactory CNS neurons starts already during embryonic and larval stages, ensuring that a prepatterned dendritic target field is established by the time ORN axons project into the antennal lobe.[31] Projection neurons (PNs) and local interneurons (LNs) originate from asymmetrically dividing neural precursor cells called neuroblasts (Fig. 7).[89] At each division neuroblasts produce serially a new neuroblast and a ganglion mother cell, which divides once more to generate two terminally differentiated neurons (Fig. 7). PNs are derived from three neuroblasts: an antero-dorsal (ad), a lateral (la) and a ventral (ve) neuroblast, corresponding to the three groups of cell bodies.[89] It has been shown that the ad and la PN lineages send dendrites to stereotyped and mutually exclusive sets of glomeruli.[12] Using the MARCM method to perform a systematic fate mapping analysis of PNs, Jefferis et al could demonstrate a direct correlation between the larval PN lineage and birth time with their dendritic targeting onto distinct glomeruli.[83] In addition, embryonic-born PNs participate in both the larval and adult olfactory circuits.[90] In the larva, these neurons generally innervate a single glomerulus in the antennal lobe and persist in the adult olfactory circuit, also prespecified by birth order to innervate a subset of glomeruli distinct from larval-born PNs. Developmental studies indicate that these neurons undergo stereotyped pruning of their dendrites and axon terminal branches locally during early metamorphosis, which requires cell-autonomous reception of the nuclear hormone ecdysone.[90]

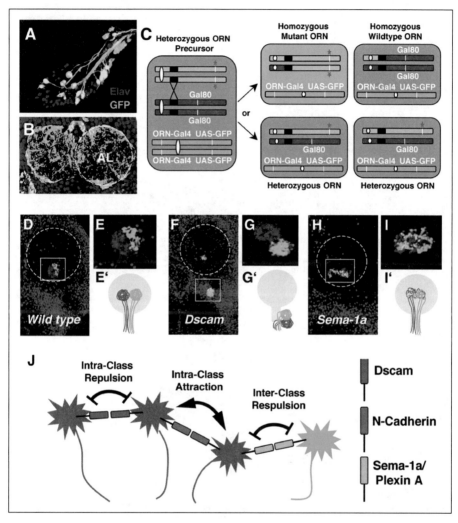

Figure 6. Analysis of gene functions involved in ORN connectivity development. A-C) Mosaic analysis in developing ORNs using the MARCM system. Induction of MARCM clones under *eyFlp* control leads to homozygous (GFP-positive) ORNs in the maxillary palps A) and antenna (not shown) and allows to follow their axonal projections into the AL (B), whereas the AL target neurons (LNs and PNs) next to the AL remain unaffected (red, GFP-negative). C) Schematic illustrating the segregation of the different chromosomes (asterisk indicates the mutation) from the heterozygous ORN precursor cell into the different daughter cells. Due to the loss of the Gal80 insertion after mitotic recombination at the FRT sites (black box), the homozygous mutant ORNs start to express GFP in a Gal4/UAS-dependent manner, whereas in homozygous wildtype or heterozygous ORNs the expression of GFP remains repressed due to the presence of Gal80. D, E, E') The projection of two ORN classes (green and red) onto neighboring glomeruli is shown. F, G, G') Loss of *Dscam* in ORN-specific MARCM clones lead to a premature convergence inside and outside the AL, but mutant axons sort out according to their OR class identity. H, I, I') Following the removal of *Semaphorin-1a* *(Sema-1a)*, mutant ORN axons project to the target region but fail to sort into class-specific glomeruli. J) Model of the inter-axonal interactions mediated by different neuronal cell surface molecules (see text).

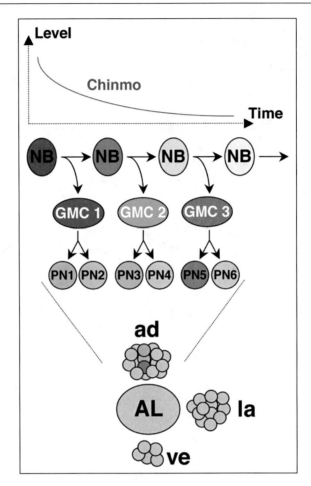

Figure 7. Generation of Projection Neurons during AL development. Projection Neurons (PNs) in each of the three PN clusters, the anterior-dorsal (ad), lateral (la) and ventral (ve) cluster, derive from a distinct neuroblast (NB). The different PN classes inside each cluster (e.g., PN1, PN2, etc.) are generated at defined time points from the dividing NB though an intermediate ganglion mother cell (GMC). Recent data indicate that the level of the POU-domain type transcription factor Chinmo in the dividing NB defines a critical determinant in the control of PN identity, with high levels giving rises to early-born PNs and low levels to late-born PNs.

How is PN diversity generated through the series of NB divisions? First insights into the molecular mechanism that lead to PN diversification came through the identification of the putative transcription factor Chinmo that confers temporal identity on the neural progeny of mushroom body and projection neurons neuroblasts (Fig. 7).[91] In the PN lineage, loss of Chinmo autonomously causes early-born neurons to adopt the fates of late-born neurons from the same lineages. Although the molecular mechanisms that control PN fate identity is not clear yet, studies in mushroom bodies indicate the generation of a temporal gradient of Chinmo (Fig. 7) through primarily posttranscriptional regulation which helps to specify distinct birth order-dependent cell fates in an extended neuronal lineage.[91]

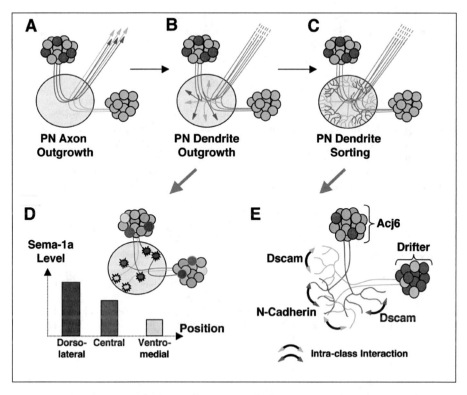

Figure 8. Development of PN connectivity. (A-C) Schematic drawings of the three main steps in PN axon and dendrite development. A) Adult PNs first send out axonal processes towards the mushroom bodies and lateral horn. B) PNs develop dendritic branches which project to different regions, according to their later glomerular position in the AL. C) Different types of inter-dendritic interactions further restrict PN dendrites to their final AL position. D) The level of Semaphorin-1a in developing PNs determines their dendrite positioning along the dorso-ventral AL axis; high levels lead to a dorso-lateral location whereas PNs expressing low Sema-1a levels project to ventro-medial positions. E) PN dendrites having reached their crude position in the AL perform different types of interactions (mediated by N-Cadherin and Dscam) to elaborate and restrict their dendritic branches.

Development of PN Dendrites

Shortly after birth during larval development, PNs extend axons along the main tracts connecting the antennal lobe to higher olfactory centres, the MB and LH, however no axonal arborizations are formed within those CNS regions (Fig. 8A).[31] At the time of larval/pupal transition, PN dendrite development starts with the extension of dendritic processes into different regions of the AL (Fig. 8B), so that by about 20 h APF spatially restricted but still overlapping dendritic arbours occupy the early AL.[31] At the same time, ORN axons have just reached the developing antennal lobe. The directional outgrowth is followed by a period of inter-dendritic interaction (Fig. 8C), resulting in a further refinement of arborization according to their PN class identity.[84] Class-specific branching of PN axons is evident in the lateral horn by 24-30 h APF.[31] Thus the PN axonal development relevant to wiring occurs relatively synchronously with dendritic development.

Recently, several molecular determinates, e.g., transcription factors and cell surface molecules, have been identified that are involved in the two main steps of PN dendrite development, directional outgrowth and class-specific sorting.[84-86,92,93] Interestingly, the same molecules described above to control ORN axon-axon interaction, Semaphorin-1a, N-Cadherin and Dscam, also have an independent function during PN dendrite patterning. Somewhat surprising came the observation that Sema-1a levels cell-autonomously direct initial PN targeting in the antennal lobe along the dorsal-lateral/ventral-medial axis (Fig. 8D).[86] This function requires the cytoplasmic domain, which could mediate signalling upon binding to a yet unknown ligand, distributed in a gradient along in the early AL to specify dendrite positioning.[86]

Mosaic analyses suggest that N-Cadherin mediates dendro-dendritic interactions between PNs and thus contributes to spatial restriction of PN dendrites thereby sharpening the boundaries between glomeruli (Fig. 8E).[84] Developmental studies reveal that the dendrites of *N-Cadherin* mutant PNs occupy the same global positions as their wild-type counterparts during early pupal development but fail to sort in a PN class specific pattern. A possible explanation for the dendritic defect is that N-Cadherin expressed on the surface of PN dendrites confers proper adhesiveness to the dendrite during and after the initial targeting event. Loss of N-Cadherin results in reduced cell adhesion, allowing dendrites to more easily invade the neighboring glomeruli. In contrast to the inhibition of dendritic extensions, Dscam acts in projection neurons and local interneurons to control the elaboration of dendritic fields (Fig. 8E).[85] The removal of Dscam selectively from PNs or LNs leads to a marked reduction in their dendritic field size whereas Dscam overexpression causes dendrites to shift their relative local position. Thus, similar to the ORN axon pattering, sequential attractive and repulsive interactions seem to mediate the final positioning of PN dendrites.

Beside the cell surface molecules directly involved in inter-dendritic communication, the functional analysis of PN-intrinsic mechanisms has led to the identification of several transcription factors (TFs) that control dendritic targeting[86,92] Members of different TF families, e.g., LIM-homeodomain TFs (Islet and Lim1), homeodomain TFs (Cut), zinc-finger TFs (Squeeze) and POU-domain TFs (Acj6 and Drifter) lead in PN-specific loss-of-function mosaic clones to either coarse or local dendrite targeting defects, suggesting that they have qualitatively different instructive information. Most of these TFs show a spatially restricted expression pattern, e.g., Acj6 and Drifter, are expressed in adPNs and laPNs respectively (Fig. 8E).[92] Misexpression experiments induces specific changes of targeting specificity suggest that PN classes are at least partially defined by combinatorial expression of TFs that regulate different steps of dendritic targeting, some specifying the coarse area (e.g., Cut), followed by others controlling local glomerular choice within the area (e.g., Drifter and Acj6).

Concluding Remarks

Initial studies in other insects and mammals have emphasized the organizing role of ORNs in AL development. For instance in *Manduca* surgical removal of the antenna prevents normal glomerular formation[94,95] and antennal disc transplantation between different sexes results in the formation of glomeruli with a morphology that is most typical of the donor sex.[96] The results in *Drosophila* presented here suggested that both ORNs and PNs have substantial autonomous patterning ability in which both neuronal types target coarsely without interacting with their partners. Experiments in which ORN axon and PN dendrite targeting are differentially affected provide first insights into the relative contribution of both synaptic partners in determining connection specificity. Cell-type specific removal of N-Cadherin from PN dendrites does not affect the site specific convergence of the partner ORNs.[84] In addition, the local shift in ORN axon convergence or PN dendrite positioning leads to the corresponding displacement of the synaptic partner, which so far is the strongest indication for a cell-type specific recognition code.[88]

Based on the cellular interactions during pupal AL development and the resulting connectivity defect following the cell-type specific mutant analysis described above we suggest the following model for ORN-PN matching (Fig. 9). The first cellular event seems to be the generation of a coarse map of PN dendrites in the developing AL (Step 1). Initial ORN axon targeting is equally imprecise. The axons of a particular ORN class reach their target area and intermingle with axons of spatially related targets. *Intra*-class axonal attraction combined with *inter*-class axonal retraction forces this local blend of different axon classes to segregate from one another (Step 2). When

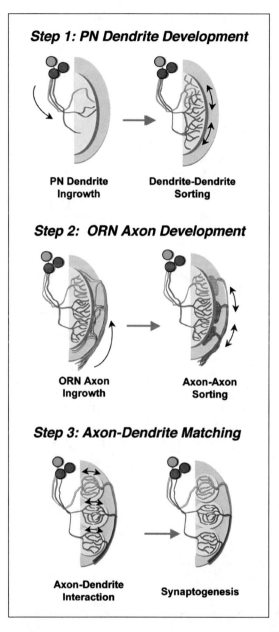

Figure 9. Model of neuronal connectivity development in the *Drosophila* olfactory system. The development of neuronal connections in the *Drosophila* AL can be divided into three consecutive steps. First, PN dendrite projection and dendro-dendritic interactions lead to prepatterned target field before ORN axons reach the AL. In a second step, ORN axons of the same OR class grow into the AL and target to the approximate position followed by axon-axon interactions in to converge into OR class specific protoglomeruli. In the final step of glomerulus formation, class-specific ORN-PN recognition leads to the restriction of axons and dendrites into single glomerular units, in which the different neuronal processes assemble into functional circuits.

a critical concentration of similar axons is reached, axonal protoglomeruli begin to form at the periphery of the antennal lobe (Step 2). In the final step, class-specific ORN-PN recognition initiates the glomerulus assembly followed by synaptogenesis and glial mediated isolation of new emerging synaptic units. Once established these synaptic units are rather stable, manipulations in the adult fly, e.g., the selective cell ablation or differential olfactory experience leads to only minor intra-glomerular changes.[76,97] Based on this model ORN axon and PN dendrite targeting are initially two separate patterning events and subsequent axon-dendrite matching is the final step by which two prepatterned fields are merged.

How the differentiation of about 50 distinct synaptic partners is coordinated remains one of the challenging questions in olfactory system research. In the peripheral olfactory system, distinct types of ORNs have to become specified and the subsequent differentiation has to be coupled to the neurogenesis within developing sensilla, the development of axon projection patterns and the eventual expression of individual odorant receptors. In the central olfactory system, the development of the dendritic projection has to be coordinated with the distinct axonal branching pattern in the higher brain centers.[33,98] The *Drosophila* olfactory system provides a powerful model to address these fundamental issues of neuroscience research.

References

1. Chklovskii DB, Koulakov AA. Maps in the brain: what can we learn from them? Annu Rev Neurosci 2004; 27:369-392.
2. Miller G. 2004 Nobel Prizes. Axel, Buck share award for deciphering how the nose knows. Science 2004; 306(5694):207.
3. Buck L, Axel R. A novel multigene family may encode odorant receptors: a molecular basis for odor recognition. Cell 1991; 65(1):175-187.
4. Chess A, Simon I, Cedar H et al. Allelic inactivation regulates olfactory receptor gene expression. Cell 1994; 78(5):823-834.
5. Vassar R, Ngai J, Axel R. Spatial segregation of odorant receptor expression in the mammalian olfactory epithelium. Cell 1993; 74(2):309-318.
6. Mombaerts P, Wang F, Dulac C et al. Visualizing an olfactory sensory map. Cell 1996; 87(4):675-686.
7. Vassar R, Chao SK, Sitcheran R et al. Topographic organization of sensory projections to the olfactory bulb. Cell 1994; 79(6):981-991.
8. Feinstein P, Bozza T, Rodriguez I et al. Axon guidance of mouse olfactory sensory neurons by odorant receptors and the beta2 adrenergic receptor. Cell 2004; 117(6):833-846.
9. Feinstein P, Mombaerts P. A contextual model for axonal sorting into glomeruli in the mouse olfactory system. Cell 2004; 117(6):817-831.
10. Imai T, Suzuki M, Sakano H. Odorant receptor-derived cAMP signals direct axonal targeting. Science 2006; 314(5799):657-661.
11. Serizawa S, Miyamichi K, Takeuchi H et al. A neuronal identity code for the odorant receptor-specific and activity-dependent axon sorting. Cell 2006; 127(5):1057-1069.
12. Stocker RF, Lienhard MC, Borst A et al. Neuronal architecture of the antennal lobe in Drosophila melanogaster. Cell Tissue Res 1990; 262(1):9-34.
13. Stocker RF. The organization of the chemosensory system in Drosophila melanogaster: a review. Cell Tissue Res 1994; 275(1):3-26.
14. Stocker RF. Drosophila as a focus in olfactory research: mapping of olfactory sensilla by fine structure, odor specificity, odorant receptor expression and central connectivity. Microsc Res Tech 2001; 55(5):284-296.
15. Stowers L. Neuronal development: specifying a hard-wired circuit. Curr Biol 2004; 14(2):R62-64.
16. Vosshall LB, Wong AM, Axel R. An olfactory sensory map in the fly brain. Cell 2000; 102(2):147-159.
17. Komiyama T, Luo L. Development of wiring specificity in the olfactory system. Curr Opin Neurobiol 2006; 16(1):67-73.
18. Jefferis GS, Marin EC, Watts RJ et al. Development of neuronal connectivity in Drosophila antennal lobes and mushroom bodies. Curr Opin Neurobiol 2002; 12(1):80-86.
19. Jefferis GS, Hummel T. Wiring specificity in the olfactory system. Semin Cell Dev Biol 2006; 17(1):50-65.
20. Clyne PJ, Warr CG, Freeman MR et al. A novel family of divergent seven-transmembrane proteins: candidate odorant receptors in Drosophila. Neuron 1999; 22(2):327-338.

21. Vosshall LB, Amrein H, Morozov PS, Rzhetsky A, Axel R. A spatial map of olfactory receptor expression in the Drosophila antenna. Cell 1999; 96(5):725-736.
22. Lomvardas S, Barnea G, Pisapia DJ et al. Interchromosomal interactions and olfactory receptor choice. Cell 2006; 126(2):403-413.
23. Ray A, van Naters WG, Shiraiwa T et al. Mechanisms of odor receptor gene choice in Drosophila. Neuron 2007; 53(3):353-369.
24. Gao Q, Yuan B, Chess A. Convergent projections of Drosophila olfactory neurons to specific glomeruli in the antennal lobe. Nat Neurosci 2000; 3(8):780-785.
25. Couto A, Alenius M, Dickson BJ. Molecular, anatomical and functional organization of the Drosophila olfactory system. Curr Biol 2005; 15(17):1535-1547.
26. Fishilevich E, Vosshall LB. Genetic and functional subdivision of the Drosophila antennal lobe. Curr Biol 2005; 15(17):1548-1553.
27. Laissue PP, Reiter C, Hiesinger PR et al. Three-dimensional reconstruction of the antennal lobe in Drosophila melanogaster. J Comp Neurol 1999; 405(4):543-552.
28. Stocker RF, Singh RN, Schorderet M et al. Projection patterns of different types of antennal sensilla in the antennal glomeruli of Drosophila melanogaster. Cell Tissue Res 1983; 232(2):237-248.
29. Jhaveri D, Saharan S, Sen A et al. Positioning sensory terminals in the olfactory lobe of Drosophila by Robo signaling. Development 2004; 131(9):1903-1912.
30. Jhaveri D, Sen A, Rodrigues V. Mechanisms underlying olfactory neuronal connectivity in Drosophila-the atonal lineage organizes the periphery while sensory neurons and glia pattern the olfactory lobe. Dev Biol 2000; 226(1):73-87.
31. Jefferis GS, Vyas RM, Berdnik D et al. Developmental origin of wiring specificity in the olfactory system of Drosophila. Development 2004; 131(1):117-130.
32. Wong AM, Wang JW, Axel R. Spatial representation of the glomerular map in the Drosophila protocerebrum. Cell 2002; 109(2):229-241.
33. Marin EC, Jefferis GS, Komiyama et al.Representation of the glomerular olfactory map in the Drosophila brain. Cell 2002; 109(2):243-255.
34. Wilson RI, Turner GC, Laurent G. Transformation of olfactory representations in the Drosophila antennal lobe. Science 2004; 303(5656):366-370.
35. Wilson RI, Laurent G. Role of GABAergic inhibition in shaping odor-evoked spatiotemporal patterns in the Drosophila antennal lobe. J Neurosci 2005; 25(40):9069-9079.
36. Olsen SR, Bhandawat V, Wilson RI. Excitatory interactions between olfactory processing channels in the Drosophila antennal lobe. Neuron 2007; 54(1):89-103.
37. Shang Y, Claridge-Chang A, Sjulson L et al. Excitatory local circuits and their implications for olfactory processing in the fly antennal lobe. Cell 2007; 128(3):601-612.
38. Distler PG, Boeckh J. An improved model of the synaptic organization of insect olfactory glomeruli. Ann NY Acad Sci 1998; 855:508-510.
39. Distler PG, Gruber C, Boeckh J. Synaptic connections between GABA-immunoreactive neurons and uniglomerular projection neurons within the antennal lobe of the cockroach, Periplaneta americana. Synapse 1998; 29(1):1-13.
40. Distler PG, Boeckh J. Synaptic connection between olfactory receptor cells and uniglomerular projection neurons in the antennal lobe of the American cockroach, Periplaneta americana. J Comp Neurol 1996; 370(1):35-46.
41. Riesgo-Escovar JR, Piekos WB, Carlson JR. The Drosophila antenna: ultrastructural and physiological studies in wild-type and lozenge mutants. J Comp Physiol [A] 1997; 180(2):151-160.
42. Shanbhag S, Muller, B, Steinbrecht A. Atlas of olffactory organs of Drosophila melanogaster: I Types, external organisation, innervation and distribution of olfactory sensilla. Int J Insect Morphol and Embryol 1999; 28:377-397.
43. Clyne PJ, Certel SJ, de Bruyne et al.The odor specificities of a subset of olfactory receptor neurons are governed by Acj6, a POU-domain transcription factor. Neuron 1999; 22(2):339-347.
44. de Bruyne M, Clyne PJ, Carlson JR. Odor coding in a model olfactory organ: the Drosophila maxillary palp. J Neurosci 1999; 19(11):4520-4532.
45. de Bruyne M, Foster K, Carlson JR. Odor coding in the Drosophila antenna. Neuron 2001; 30(2):537-552.
46. Elmore T, Ignell R, Carlson JR et al. Targeted mutation of a Drosophila odor receptor defines receptor requirement in a novel class of sensillum. J Neurosci 2003; 23(30):9906-9912.
47. Yao CA, Ignell R, Carlson JR. Chemosensory coding by neurons in the coeloconic sensilla of the Drosophila antenna. J Neurosci 2005; 25(37):8359-8367.
48. van der Goes van Naters W, Carlson JR. Receptors and neurons for fly odors in Drosophila. Curr Biol 2007; 17(7):606-612.

49. Haynie JL, Bryant PJ. Development of the eye-antenna imaginal disc and morphogenesis of the adult head in Drosophila melanogaster. J Exp Zool 1986; 237(3):293-308.
50. Cohen SM, Di Nardo S. Wingless: from embryo to adult. Trends Genet 1993; 9(6):189-192.
51. Jhaveri D, Sen A, Reddy GV et al. Sense organ identity in the Drosophila antenna is specified by the expression of the proneural gene atonal. Mech Dev 2000; 99(1-2):101-111.
52. Gomez-Skarmeta JL, Campuzano S, Modolell J. Half a century of neural prepatterning: the story of a few bristles and many genes. Nat Rev Neurosci 2003; 4(7):587-598.
53. Kiefer JC, Jarman A, Johnson J. Proneural factors and neurogenesis. Dev Dyn 2005; 234(3):808-813.
54. Goulding SE, zur Lage P, Jarman AP. amos, a proneural gene for Drosophila olfactory sense organs that is regulated by lozenge. Neuron 2000; 25(1):69-78.
55. Gupta BP, Rodrigues V. Atonal is a proneural gene for a subset of olfactory sense organs in Drosophila. Genes Cells 1997; 2(3):225-233.
56. Jan YN, Jan LY. Neuronal cell fate specification in Drosophila. Curr Opin Neurobiol 1994; 4(1):8-13.
57. Reddy GV, Gupta B, Ray K et al. Development of the Drosophila olfactory sense organs utilizes cell-cell interactions as well as lineage. Development 1997; 124(3):703-712.
58. Ray K, Rodrigues V. Cellular events during development of the olfactory sense organs in Drosophila melanogaster. Dev Biol 1995; 167(2):426-438.
59. zur Lage PI, Prentice DR, Holohan EE et al. The Drosophila proneural gene amos promotes olfactory sensillum formation and suppresses bristle formation. Development 2003; 130(19):4683-4693.
60. Gupta BP, Flores GV, Banerjee U et al. Patterning an epidermal field: Drosophila lozenge, a member of the AML-1/Runt family of transcription factors, specifies olfactory sense organ type in a dose-dependent manner. Dev Biol 1998; 203(2):400-411.
61. Venkatesh SS, Sensilla RN on the third antennal segment of Drosophila melanogaster Meigen (Diptera: Drosophilidae). Int J Insect Morphol Embryol 1984; 13:51-63.
62. Lienhard MC, Stocker RF. The development of the sensory neuron pattern in the antennal disc of wild-type and mutant (lz3, ssa) Drosophila melanogaster. Development 1991; 112(4):1063-1075.
63. Sen A, Reddy GV, Rodrigues V. Combinatorial expression of Prospero, Seven-up and Elav identifies progenitor cell types during sense-organ differentiation in the Drosophila antenna. Dev Biol 2003; 254(1):79-92.
64. Endo K, Aoki T, Yoda Y, Kimura K et al. Notch signal organizes the Drosophila olfactory circuitry by diversifying the sensory neuronal lineages. Nat Neurosci 2007; 10(2):153-160.
65. Lee T, Luo L. Mosaic analysis with a repressible cell marker (MARCM) for Drosophila neural development. Trends Neurosci 2001; 24(5):251-254.
66. Lee T, Luo L. Mosaic analysis with a repressible cell marker for studies of gene function in neuronal morphogenesis. Neuron 1999; 22(3):451-461.
67. Manning L, Doe CQ. Prospero distinguishes sibling cell fate without asymmetric localization in the Drosophila adult external sense organ lineage. Development 1999; 126(10):2063-2071.
68. Reddy GV, Rodrigues V. Sibling cell fate in the Drosophila adult external sense organ lineage is specified by prospero function, which is regulated by Numb and Notch. Development 1999; 126(10):2083-2092.
69. Guo M, Bier E, Jan LY, et al. tramtrack acts downstream of numb to specify distinct daughter cell fates during asymmetric cell divisions in the Drosophila PNS. Neuron 1995; 14(5):913-925.
70. Jan YN, Jan LY. Asymmetric cell division. Nature 1998; 392(6678):775-778.
71. Gho M, Bellaiche Y, Schweisguth F. Revisiting the Drosophila microchaete lineage: a novel intrinsically asymmetric cell division generates a glial cell. Development 1999; 126(16):3573-3584.
72. Jhaveri D, Rodrigues V. Sensory neurons of the Atonal lineage pioneer the formation of glomeruli within the adult Drosophila olfactory lobe. Development 2002; 129(5):1251-1260.
73. Sen A, Shetty C, Jhaveri D et al. Distinct types of glial cells populate the Drosophila antenna. BMC Dev Biol 2005; 5:25.
74. Hummel T, Zipursky SL. Afferent induction of olfactory glomeruli requires N-cadherin. Neuron 2004; 42(1):77-88.
75. Sweeney LB, Couto A, Chou YH et al. Temporal target restriction of olfactory receptor neurons by Semaphorin-1a/PlexinA-mediated axon-axon interactions. Neuron 2007; 53(2):185-200.
76. Devaud JM, Acebes A, Ramaswami M et al. Structural and functional changes in the olfactory pathway of adult Drosophila take place at a critical age. J Neurobiol 2003; 56(1):13-23.
77. Bhalerao S, Sen A, Stocker R et al. Olfactory neurons expressing identified receptor genes project to subsets of glomeruli within the antennal lobe of Drosophila melanogaster. J Neurobiol 2003; 54(4):577-592.
78. Mombaerts P. Axonal wiring in the mouse olfactory system. Annu Rev Cell Dev Biol 2006; 22:713-737.

79. Tolbert LP, Oland LA. A role for glia in the development of organized neuropilar structures. Trends Neurosci 1989; 12(2):70-75.
80. Rossler W, Oland LA, Higgins MR et al. Development of a glia-rich axon-sorting zone in the olfactory pathway of the moth Manduca sexta. J Neurosci 1999; 19(22):9865-9877.
81. Hummel T, Vasconcelos ML, Clemens JC et al. Axonal targeting of olfactory receptor neurons in Drosophila is controlled by Dscam. Neuron 2003; 37(2):221-231.
82. Komiyama T, Carlson JR, Luo L. Olfactory receptor neuron axon targeting: intrinsic transcriptional control and hierarchical interactions. Nat Neurosci 2004; 7(8):819-825.
83. Jefferis GS, Marin EC, Stocker RF et al. Target neuron prespecification in the olfactory map of Drosophila. Nature 2001; 414(6860):204-208.
84. Zhu H, Luo L. Diverse functions of N-cadherin in dendritic and axonal terminal arborization of olfactory projection neurons. Neuron 2004; 42(1):63-75.
85. Zhu H, Hummel T, Clemens JC et al. Dendritic patterning by Dscam and synaptic partner matching in the Drosophila antennal lobe. Nat Neurosci 2006; 9(3):349-355.
86. Komiyama T, Luo L. Intrinsic control of precise dendritic targeting by an ensemble of transcription factors. Curr Biol 2007; 17(3):278-285.
87. Ang LH, Kim J, Stepensky V et alDock and Pak regulate olfactory axon pathfinding in Drosophila. Development 2003; 130(7):1307-1316.
88. Lattemann M, Zierau A, Schulte C et al. Semaphorin-1a controls receptor neuron-specific axonal convergence in the primary olfactory center of Drosophila. Neuron 2007; 53(2):169-184.
89. Stocker RF, Heimbeck G, Gendre N et al. Neuroblast ablation in Drosophila P[GAL4] lines reveals origins of olfactory interneurons. J Neurobiol 1997; 32(5):443-456.
90. Marin EC, Watts RJ, Tanaka NK et al. Developmentally programmed remodeling of the Drosophila olfactory circuit. Development 2005; 132(4):725-737.
91. Zhu S, Lin S, Kao CF et al. Gradients of the Drosophila Chinmo BTB-zinc finger protein govern neuronal temporal identity. Cell 2006; 127(2):409-422.
92. Komiyama T, Johnson WA, Luo L et al. From lineage to wiring specificity. POU domain transcription factors control precise connections of Drosophila olfactory projection neurons. Cell 2003; 112(2):157-167.
93. Komiyama T, Sweeney LB, Schuldiner O et al. Graded expression of semaphorin-1a cell-autonomously directs dendritic targeting of olfactory projection neurons. Cell 2007; 128(2):399-410.
94. Tolbert LP, Sirianni PA. Requirement for olfactory axons in the induction and stabilization of olfactory glomeruli in an insect. J Comp Neurol 1990; 298(1):69-82.
95. Oland LA, Orr G, Tolbert LP. Construction of a protoglomerular template by olfactory axons initiates the formation of olfactory glomeruli in the insect brain. J Neurosci 1990; 10(7):2096-2112.
96. Rossler W, Randolph PW, Tolbert LP et al. Axons of olfactory receptor cells of transsexually grafted antennae induce development of sexually dimorphic glomeruli in Manduca sexta. J Neurobiol 1999; 38(4):521-541.
97. Berdnik D, Chihara T, Couto A et al. Wiring stability of the adult Drosophila olfactory circuit after lesion. J Neurosci 2006; 26(13):3367-3376.
98. Jefferis GS, Potter CJ, Chan AM et al. Comprehensive maps of Drosophila higher olfactory centers: spatially segregated fruit and pheromone representation. Cell 2007; 128(6):1187-1203.

CHAPTER 7

The Olfactory Sensory Map in *Drosophila*

Philippe P. Laissue and Leslie B. Vosshall*

Abstract

The fruit fly (*Drosophila melanogaster*) exhibits robust odor-evoked behaviors in response to cues from diverse host plants and pheromonal cues from other flies. Understanding how the adult olfactory system supports the perception of these odorous chemicals and translates them into appropriate attraction or avoidance behaviors is an important goal in contemporary sensory neuroscience. Recent advances in genomics and molecular neurobiology have provided an unprecedented level of detail into how the adult *Drosophila* olfactory system is organized. Volatile odorants are sensed by two bilaterally symmetric olfactory sensory appendages, the third segment of the antenna and the maxillary palps, which respectively contain approximately 1200 and 120 olfactory sensory neurons (OSNs) each. These OSNs express a divergent family of seven transmembrane domain odorant receptors (ORs) with no homology to vertebrate ORs, which determine the odor specificity of a given OSN. *Drosophila* was the first animal for which all OR genes were cloned, their patterns of gene expression determined and axonal projections of most OSNs elucidated. In vivo electrophysiology has been used to decode the ligand response profiles of most of the ORs, providing insight into the initial logic of olfactory coding in the fly. This chapter will review the molecular biology, neuroanatomy and function of the peripheral olfactory system of *Drosophila*.

Introduction

Sensory systems—touch, hearing, vision, taste, smell—map features of the external world into internal representations in the brain that ultimately allow all animals to navigate their environments. The physical senses of touch and vision use topographic mapping approaches to represent discrete dimensions of the external world. For example, the visual system uses retinotopic mapping to organize the field of view in the lateral geniculate nucleus, such that there is an orderly representation of the visual field in the brain.[1] The somatosensory system uses somatotopic mapping to project not the external world but the body plan onto the somatosensory cortex.[2,3] Thus it is not the environment per se that is mapped, but the various parts of the body, allowing an animal to determine with precision where it is being touched by a physical stimulus. The auditory system maps sound frequencies along a tonotopic axis in the cochlea and the auditory cortex, allowing sound to be broken into its component parts and later synthesized into a coherent representation of what was heard.[4,5] An important feature of the auditory system is the precision by which it permits animals to localize sound in space. This is accomplished by central brain comparisons of input into the left and right ears. These mapping approaches allow visual, somatosensory and auditory cortex to represent important features of visual, mechanical and auditory stimuli and relate them to physical space in the external world.

*Corresponding Author: Leslie B. Vosshall—Laboratory of Neurogenetics and Behavior, The Rockefeller University, 1230 York Avenue, Box 63, New York, New York 10021, USA. Email: leslie@mail.rockefeller.edu

Brain Development in Drosophila melanogaster, edited by Gerhard M. Technau.
©2008 Landes Bioscience and Springer Science+Business Media.

The chemical senses—taste and smell—are less well understood than the physical senses but appear to use a different strategy to represent gustatory and olfactory cues encountered in the environment. Instead of mapping primarily the position of the external stimulus and its relationship to the individual, the gustatory and olfactory systems categorize the identity and quality of the stimulus. The tongue can detect at least five different taste qualities—bitter, sweet, sour, salty and umami, the taste of monosodium glutamate. Insects appear to have all of these taste qualities, with the possible exception of umami and the addition of a "water" sense.[6,7] Each of these taste qualities is perceived by structurally and functionally discrete gustatory neurons in the tongue of vertebrates[8] and labial palps of insects.[6,9] It is still unclear in the field whether these taste qualities remain segregated into stimulus-specific labeled lines from the periphery to higher brain centers,[8,10,11] or whether distributed coding across groups of sensory and central brain neurons allows animals to distinguish tastes of different modalities such as bitter and sweet.[12,13] There is clear evidence in *Drosophila* that pathways for bitter and sweet tastes are anatomically and functionally separate senses that elicit innate aversive and appetitive responses, respectively.[9-11]

The olfactory system is capable of detecting an extremely large number of volatile chemical stimuli, possibly exceeding tens of thousands, although the total olfactory coding capacity of any animal has never been exhaustively catalogued.[14] The ability to recognize such a vast number of odorous ligands is thought to be due to the special properties of the ORs, the large family of membrane proteins that is selectively expressed in OSNs in the olfactory epithelium of vertebrates and antennae of insects. ORs have selective but broad ligand-binding properties, such that a given OR is activated by multiple odors and a given odor activates multiple ORs.[15-18] This combinatorial coding strategy based on a large family of ORs with broad but selective ligand pharmacology in part accounts for the ability of animals to detect and discriminate a number of odors that far exceeds the number of ORs they possess.

In all arthropods and vertebrates studied to date, the early olfactory system is organized into a large number of spherical neuropil elements, called glomeruli.[19,20] Olfactory glomeruli represent points of convergence where OSNs expressing the same OR synapse with inhibitory local interneurons and secondary neurons that relay olfactory information to higher brain centers.[21-25] There is some evidence in mammals that the olfactory system maps odor stimuli along a chemotopic axis in the vertebrate olfactory bulb.[26-28] Thus neurons responsive to odors sharing an alcohol functional group will tend to innervate adjacent regions in the bulb and these regions appear to be organized by carbon chain length.[26,27] This type of chemotopy is less apparent in insect systems.[29-32]

This chapter will review recent progress in our understanding of the organization and function of the adult *Drosophila* olfactory system. The accompanying chapter by Veronica Rodrigues and Thomas Hummel will address the development and early patterning of the olfactory system. The accompanying chapter by Reinhard Stocker concerns the unique organization of the larval olfactory system.

Olfactory Organs and Olfactory Sensory Neurons of *Drosophila*

Fruit flies detect odors through two olfactory sensory organs on the head, the antenna and maxillary palp (Fig. 1). These olfactory appendages are covered with a large number of sensory hairs, called sensilla, which house and protect the underlying OSNs that are specialized to detect odors. Olfactory sensilla can be distinguished morphologically from thermo- and hygro-sensitive sensilla by the presence of a large number of small pores that perforate the shaft of the sensillum and which are believed to allow access to odors (reviewed in ref. 33). A total of about 410 olfactory sensilla cover the antenna, while the maxillary palp has about 60 olfactory sensilla. These hairs can be divided into three distinct morphological and functional classes: Club-shaped basiconic sensilla, long and pointed trichoid sensilla and short, peg-shaped coeloconic sensilla (Fig. 1).

Further morphological and functional distinctions subdivide both basiconic and trichoid sensilla into additional subclasses, which differ by the size and density of odor pores, the number of neurons housed in each sensillum and their distribution on the antenna (Fig. 1)[29,33-36] The different sensilla types are distributed in a highly stereotyped fashion over the surface of the antenna. Large basiconic sensilla are clustered at the medial face of the antenna, while the three types of trichoid sensilla are arranged in diagonal bands across the lateral face of the antenna (Fig. 1).

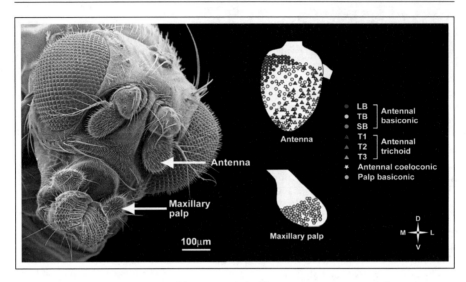

Figure 1. Peripheral organization of the *Drosophila* olfactory system. Scanning electron micrograph of a *Drosophila* head indicating the two major sensory organs, the third segment of the antenna and the maxillary palp. At right is a schematic of sensilla types and relative locations on both organs. Abbreviations: LB, large basiconic sensilla; TB, thin basiconic sensilla; SB, small basiconic sensilla; T1-T3, three different types of trichoid sensilla. SEM image by J.Scott and R.Bhatnagar, AMF, Biological Sciences, University of Alberta. Reprinted with permission from J. Scott ©2006 Biological Sciences. Cartoons adapted with permission from: Couto A, Alenius M, Dickson B. Curr Biol 2005; 15:1535-1547. ©2005 Elsevier Press.

Coeloconic sensilla are interspersed with other sensilla types, but are concentrated at the central face of the antenna. The relative position of these sensilla is well conserved as are the number of neurons innervating a given sensillum. Trichoid sensilla are named T1, T2 and T3 and contain one, two, or three OSNs, respectively. Most basiconic sensilla house two neurons, although there are several cases of four neurons per basiconic sensillum.[29,33,36] Coeloconic sensilla typically have two or three neurons. Thus the third segment of the antenna is marked by a reproducibly ordered array of olfactory sensilla that house defined and stereotyped numbers of OSNs. This patterning arises through the interplay of a cascade of patterning genes that act early in development and is discussed in the accompanying chapter by Hummel and Rodrigues.[37-40]

The maxillary palp is a simpler olfactory organ, containing fewer OSNs housed in a smaller number of basiconic sensilla. Approximately sixty basiconic sensilla each housing two OSNs can be found in this organ. Although these sensilla are externally similar, Shanbhag et al used electron microscopic analysis of OSN terminal dendrite branching in the maxillary palp to further subdivide palp sensilla into three subtypes, PB-I, PB-II and PB-III.[36] PB-I OSNs contain highly branched terminal dendrites, while PB-II OSNs are characterized by ribbon-shaped dendrites. PB-III OSNs are rarer on the palp and have an unusual thick, hollow dendritic segment. The extent to which these ultrastructural differences in antennal and maxillary palp sensilla and OSNs have functional implications will be discussed below.

Odorant Receptor Gene Expression

In vertebrates, ORs were first identified in 1991 as a very large family of related genes encoding members of the G protein-coupled receptor (GPCR) superfamily, which couples ligand binding to production of cAMP second messenger signaling.[41] During the 1990s, efforts by multiple investigators to find homologues of vertebrate ORs in insect genomes failed. In 1999 three groups used a combination of difference cloning[42] and mining of genome databases for multi-transmembrane domain proteins[42-44] to identify candidate *Drosophila* ORs. There are a total of 62 ORs, encoded by a family of 60 genes through alternative splicing.[45] The fly OR genes encode a highly divergent family of membrane-associated proteins that are selectively expressed in *Drosophila* OSNs.[42-44] These proteins are predicted to contain seven transmembrane domains, but contain no obvious homology to vertebrate ORs or the GPCR superfamily.[42,46,47] Two recent reports that looked at the membrane topology of the fly OR gene family suggested that these proteins adopt an orientation in the membrane that is inverted relative to GPCRs, such that the N-terminus faces the cytosol.[46,47] Benton et al[46] provided experimental evidence to support this atypical topology, calling into question the general assumption that fly ORs are classic GPCRs. Furthermore, different members of the fly OR family show considerably less homology to each other than most vertebrate ORs, leading to the hypothesis that this is a rapidly evolving gene family.[45]

Detailed information about the expression of each *Drosophila* OR gene is now available. Initially, RNA in situ hybridization was used to examine in which tissue and in which OSNs a given OR is expressed.[42-44] In these early papers, it was already obvious that there is a segregation of gene expression between the two major appendages: ORs expressed in the antenna are not expressed in the maxillary palp and vice versa. A later study that examined a group of 57 fly ORs confirmed this initial impression of segregation in OR repertoire between antenna (Table 1) and palp (Table 2). These appendages express non-overlapping subsets of 32 and seven OR genes, respectively (Fig. 2).[25] Two recent papers[29,30] that monitored OR gene expression with transgenic reporter techniques bring the total number of antennal-specific genes to 40 and maxillary palp-specific genes to seven. The remaining OR genes are not detectably expressed in the adult and are now known to encode the larval ORs, as discussed in the accompanying chapter by Reinhard Stocker.[48,49]

Each OR gene is expressed in a small subset of the OSNs in either olfactory organ, which varies from two to 50 OSNs per OR. The relative position and number of OR-expressing OSNs is bilaterally symmetric in the two appendages and highly stereotyped between individual flies. Early reports discussed the existence of "zones" of OR gene expression, reminiscent of the zones of OR gene expression on the olfactory turbinates of the rodent.[50,51] Careful examination of the relationship between OR gene expression and sensilla type has revealed that there is a nearly perfect correlation between the expression of OR genes and subsets of morphologically distinct basiconic, trichoid and coeloconic sensilla (Table 1).[29,52] Thus the same developmental pathways that specify the morphology of the sensilla must also dictate the numbers and functional properties of the OSNs and the specific ORs they express.

There are two unusual features of OR gene expression in *Drosophila* that set this system apart from the vertebrate paradigm, in which each OSN expresses only a single OR gene.[16,53] First, each *Drosophila* OSN expresses a broadly expressed member of the OR gene family called *Or83b*, which associates with ORs and is necessary for the proper ciliary targeting and function of all OR genes.[46,54,55] Second, a given OSN can co-express up to three conventional ORs mediating ligand selectivity along with the *Or83b* co-receptor.[29,30,56] Thus mechanisms of OR gene choice are likely to be different in the fly compared to the mouse and the feedback system that limits vertebrate OSNs to express only a single OR allele does not operate in *Drosophila*.

Ligand Tuning Profiles

What types of odors activate fly ORs and OSNs? Extracellular electrophysiological recordings that take advantage of the electrical isolation of neurons housed in a given sensillum have been a powerful tool to answer this question. Such single sensillum recordings were used to define the complete olfactory profile of the maxillary palp[57] and the majority of basiconic[58] and coeloconic[59] sensilla on the antenna. The tuning of trichoid sensilla is less well studied, but T1 sensilla are thought to respond to the aggregation pheromone cis-vaccenyl acetate.[34,60]

From these initial electrophysiological experiments, it became clear that the morphological differences in the olfactory sensilla are reflected in functional differences of the OSNs that are housed in the sensilla (Fig. 2). There is now excellent evidence that basiconic sensilla are specialized to detect food odors, both in the antenna and maxillary palp (Fig. 2, Tables 1 and 2). Trichoid

Table 1. Molecular and functional organization of the **Drosophila** *antenna*

	Antenna			
			Odors Evoking Responses (of 110 Tested)^	
OR	**Neuron**	**Glomerulus**	**+(−)**	**Strongest Ligand**
Or2a	at3	DA4m	0 (5)	no strong ligand
Or7a	ab4A	DL5	19 (30)	E2-hexenal
Or9a	ab8	VM3	21 (0)	2-pentanol
Gr10a	ab1D	DL1		
Or10a	ab1D	DL1	9 (27)	ethyl benzoate
Or13a	ai1	DC2		
Or19a	at3	DC1	6 (26)	1-octen-3-ol
Or19b	at3	DC1		
Gr21a	ab1C	V		carbon dioxide
Or22a	ab3A	DM2	29 (0)	methyl hexanoate
Or22b	ab3A	DM2		
Or23a	at2	DA3	0 (22)	no strong ligand
Or33a		DA2		
Or33b	ab5B+ab2B	DM3+DM5	0 (6)	no strong ligand
Or35a	ac1	VC3l	28 (14)	1-hexanol
Or42b	ab1	DM1		
Or43a	at3	DA4l	1 (34)	1-hexanol
Or43b	ab8A	VM2	14 (0)	ethyl butyrate
Or47a	ab5B	DM3	11 (0)	propyl acetate
Or47b	at4	VA1m+l	0 (37)	no strong ligand
Or49a	ab10	DL4		
Or49b	ab6B	VA5	3 (19)	2-methylphenol
Or56a	ab4B	DA2		
Or59b	ab2A	DM4	6 (0)	methyl acetate
Or65a	at4	DL3	0 (3)	no strong ligand
Or65b	at4	DL3		
Or65c	at4	DL3		
Or67a	ab10	DM6	31 (6)	phenylethyl alcohol
Or67b	ab9	VA3		
Or67c	ab7	VC3m	8 (9)	ethyl lactate
Or67d	at1	DA1		
Or69aA	ab9	D		
Or69aB	ab9	D		
Or82a	ab5A	VA6	1 (5)	geranyl acetate
Or83c	at2	DC3		
Or85a	ab2B	DM5	4 (31)	ethyl 3-hydroxybutyrate
Or85b	ab3B	VM5d*	22 (1)	6-methyl-5-hepten-2-one
Or85f	ab10	DL4	0 (4)	no strong ligand
Or88a	at4	VA1d	0 (11)	no strong ligand
Or92a	ab1	VA2		
Or98a	ab7A	VM5v	21 (8)	ethyl benzoate
Or98b	ab6B*	VM5d*		

*tentative; ^from Hallem and Carlson 2006; + =# odors eliciting activation of > 100 spikes/second of 110 tested; − =# odors eliciting inhibition of > −10 spikes/second of 110 tested. Data from references 29, 30, 32, 58.

Table 2. Molecular and functional organization of the Drosophila maxillary palp

			Maxillary Palp
OR	Neuron	Glomerulus	Odors Evoking Strong Responses (of 10 odors)
Or33c	pb2A	VC1	ethyl acetate, cyclohexanone, (–) fenchone
Or42a	pb1A	VM7	ethyl acetate, isoamyl acetate, E2-hexenal, cyclohexanone, 2-heptanone
Or46aA	pb2B	VA7l	4-methyl phenol
Or59c	pb3A	1	\<none\>
Or71a	pb1B	VC2	4-methyl phenol
Or85d	pb3B	VA4	isoamyl acetate, 2-heptanone
Or85e	pb2A	VC1	ethyl acetate, cyclohexanone, (–) fenchone

Data from references 29, 30, 56.

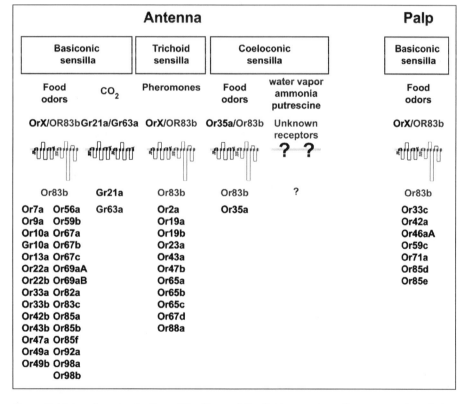

Figure 2. Molecular organization of the *Drosophila* olfactory system. Gene expression of chemosensory receptors responding to different classes of ligands is indicated. Co-receptors are listed in gray. *Gr21a* and *Gr63a* comprise the CO_2 receptor; it is not clear if either or both serve a co-receptor function. With the exception of *Or35a/Or83b* the coeloconic chemosensory receptors are still unknown. Data from references 30, 54, 56, 58-60 and 65-67.

sensilla, as observed for other insects, appear to be specialized for detecting pheromones (Fig. 2, Table 1).[34, 60-63] The coeloconic sensilla appear to detect special chemical ligands, including water vapor, ammonia and putrescine (Fig. 2, Table 2).[59] Thus the morphological differences between these sensilla types catalogued by neuroanatomists relate directly to the ligands that the underlying OSNs detect.

To determine the explicit relationship between an OR and the ligands that activate it, Carlson and co-workers developed an in vivo preparation that allows them to screen large number of ORs for their ligand response properties.[17,32,56,64] This preparation involves the Δhalo mutant, which lacks *Or22a/b* but retains expression of the *Or83b* co-receptor.[64] Different ORs can be expressed by transgenic techniques in this "empty neuron" and the OR response profile measured directly without interference from the resident OR. This technique has been used successfully to deorphanize all six classes of maxillary palp OSNs and assign specific ORs to functionally identified OSNs (Table 2).[56,57] Twenty four antennal ORs were similarly examined for their ligand specificity and most were linked to identified sensilla types.[17,29,32] A diversity of different response types for different ORs was uncovered in this work. First, some ORs are very narrowly tuned to a small number of odors, while others are broadly tuned and respond to a large number of the odorants tested (Tables 1 and 2). Second, ORs can show both excitatory and inhibitory responses to a panel of odors. Third, trichoid sensilla tend to show strong inhibitory responses and negligible excitatory responses to a large panel of general odors (Table 1),[17,32] perhaps because the native ligands for these ORs are unidentified *Drosophila* pheromones. In support of this hypothesis, *Or67d* expressed in T1 sensilla has recently been proposed as a candidate cis-vaccenyl acetate receptor.[60]

There is one conspicuous case in the antenna of a very narrowly tuned neuron, defined as ab1C. This OSN is activated selectively by and is extremely sensitive to carbon dioxide (CO_2).[58,65] These CO_2-responsive neurons co-express *Gr21a* and *Gr63a*, two of three gustatory receptor (GR) genes expressed in the antenna that may subserve an olfactory instead of a gustatory function[66,67] (Fig. 2). In fact, these two chemosensory receptors have recently been shown to mediate CO2 detection in *Drosophila*.[67]

These deorphanization efforts have lead to the conclusion that *Drosophila* ORs mediate all aspects of the odor responses in a given OSN. They determine the ligand specificity, the level of spontaneous firing of the OSN, whether an odorant will elicit excitatory or inhibitory firing patterns and the odor-evoked response dynamics.

A Receptor-Based Map of Glomerular Projections

How are axonal projections from thousands of OSNs expressing combinatorials of 47 ORs and 2 GRs organized in the antennal lobe, the insect homologue of the vertebrate olfactory bulb? The *Drosophila* antennal lobe is composed of well over 40 morphologically identifiable glomeruli whose sizes, shapes and positions are strongly conserved between different animals.[68] Genetic tools in *Drosophila* have permitted the elucidation of a nearly complete map of projections from peripheral olfactory organs to these glomeruli (Figs. 3 and 4; Tables 1 and 2).[21,25,29,30] This was achieved by expression of the OR genes to mark distinct subpopulations of OSNs with green fluorescent protein, which could be followed from the peripheral sensory appendages to the first olfactory synapse in the antennal lobe (Fig. 3).

A number of important conclusions concerning this olfactory sensory map were reached in these studies. All OSNs expressing a unique combinatorial of ORs target a single antennal lobe glomerulus. This innervation pattern is bilaterally symmetric and invariant between different animals. There is broad agreement on the assignment of OR-expressing OSNs to glomeruli named solely by neuroanatomical criteria in an earlier study.[68] A few exceptions are worth noting. Couto et al[29] referred to the glomerulus receiving projections from *Or47b* neurons as VA1v, while Fishilevich and Vosshall[30] referred to the original name for this compartmentalized glomerulus, VA1m+l,[68] which we also use in this chapter. *Or67c* was previously mapped to VC4, which we suggest is more correctly mapped to VC3m. Fishilevich and Vosshall were unable to assign the *Or46a* glomerulus,[30] while Couto et al assigned this as VA7l.[29] Finally, *Or59c* was assigned to a glomerulus named "1",[29] which appears to be a new glomerulus that was never formally named (Fig. 4).[68]

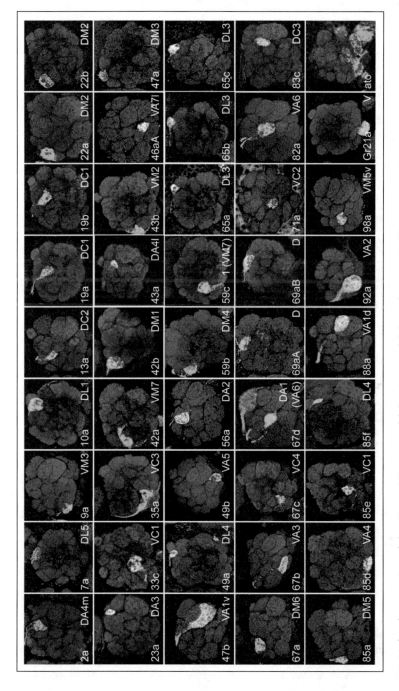

Figure 3. Molecular mapping of the *Drosophila* antennal lobe. Antennal lobes of transgenic flies carrying OR-mCD8-GFP reporters stained with anti-GFP (green) and the general neuropil marker nc82 (magenta).[68] Frontal confocal images are aligned with dorsal up and lateral right. Both Or59c and Or67d reporters label an ectopic glomerulus (in parentheses) which results from ectopic expression of the promoter in other OSNs. The lower right panel represents coeloconic glomeruli marked by expression of the *atonal* Gal4 line. Data from references.[29] Reprinted with permission from: Couto A, Alenius M, Dickson B. Curr Biol 2005; 15:1535-1547. ©2005 Elsevier Press.

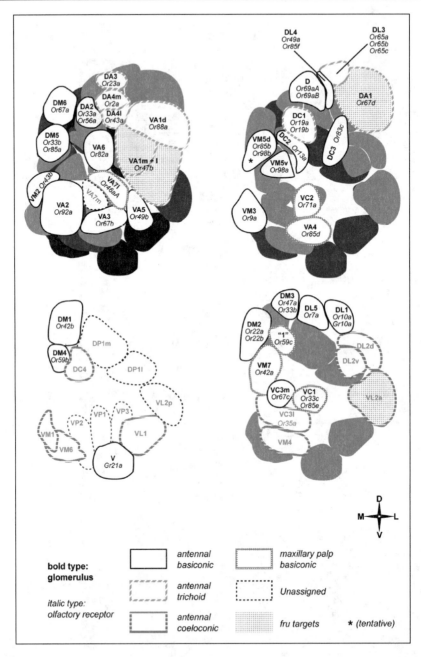

Figure 4. Molecular and anatomical map of the *Drosophila* antennal lobe. Schematic of the antennal lobe presented as frontal sections from anterior to posterior, organized clockwise from top left. Glomeruli are depth-coded with black for deep, gray for intermediate and white for superficial sections. Glomeruli are coded according to sensillum type, chemosensory organ and whether or not they are innervated by *fruitless*-positive neurons. Data from references 29, 30, 63, 66 and 68. Adapted with permission from: Fishilevich E, Vosshall LB. Curr Biol 2005; 15:1548-1553. ©2005 Elsevier Press.

We synthesize the conclusions reached in these disparate studies and present a complete map of the antennal lobe, indicating both the neuroanatomical and molecular name for each glomerulus in Figure 4. The antennal lobe comprises a total of 42 glomeruli, of which seven are subdivided into two compartments and one into three. While compartments were discovered on a purely morphological basis,[68] many have since been shown to express a single OR and due to these findings, compartments have been revealed in formerly undivided glomeruli. On a functional level, the antennal lobe can thus be said to have a total of 51 glomeruli. By including glomeruli VP1-3, the total number of glomeruli in the AL of *Drosophila* amounts to 54 glomeruli. While VP1-3 are visible in staining using synaptotagmin antibody,[61] they are not discernible with the monoclonal antibody nc82.[25,29,30,68] This may be due at least partly to their posterior-most location deep into the brain, where also the other glomeruli unassigned to ORs lie. Glomeruli in the antennal lobe are clustered into arrays, reflecting the bundling of sensilla types on the antenna and the maxillary palp. The glomeruli being connected with the maxillary palp are found predominantly in central positions, distinct from the glomeruli connected to the antenna. Antennal coeloconic OSNs project mainly to the posterior face of the antennal lobe, while antennal basiconic OSNs project to medial anterior regions of the antennal lobe. Trichoid OSNs project to the group of large glomeruli that lie at the extreme lateral regions of the antennal lobe. While these arrays have a fairly fixed design, there is no evidence for a topographic point-to-point mapping from the antenna to the antennal lobe. A direct correlation exists though between the size of a glomerulus and the number of OSNs projecting to it. For instance, *Or47b* is expressed in approximately 50 OSNs and marks a large glomerulus, VA1m+l, while *Or22a* is expressed in approximately 25 OSNs and marks a small glomerulus, DM2.

How accurate is this olfactory sensory map? Because these maps were generated with genetic reagents, it is important that the transgenic marker expression recapitulates the expression patterns of the endogenous genes. In most cases, this has been verified. Expression of the transgene, closely matching RNA in situ hybridization of the endogenous OR has been demonstrated for most published OR-Gal4 transgenes.[21,25,29,30] Nevertheless, the transgenic approach has led to some variability in glomerular mapping that almost certainly reflects artefacts of the transgenic lines themselves. For instance, both early reports of *Or23a*-expressing OSNs showed that these target two glomeruli in the antennal lobe.[21,25] Subsequent analysis of these same transgenes showed that OSNs expressing *Or23a* innervate only one of the two original glomeruli.[29,30] Ectopic expression of both *Or59c* and *Or67d* was observed, such that both transgenic reagents label one authentic and one ectopic glomerulus.[21,25] Sporadic cases of these transgenic reagents labeling multiple glomeruli have also been reported and these are almost certainly due to ectopic expression of the transgenes induced by position and other genetic background effects.[52] Another possible explanation for variation in the olfactory map is that despite the highly conserved anatomy of the antennal lobe, additional or missing glomeruli and compartments are observed between individual flies, suggesting a moderate plasticity of the olfactory system on the individual level.[29,68] Despite this inherent limitation of the genetic reagents, they have proven to be powerful tools that allowed investigators to describe the molecular neuroanatomy of the antennal lobe in unprecedented detail.

Sexual Dimorphism in the *Drosophila* Olfactory System

One further outcome of the molecular mapping of the antennal lobe was that it allowed the identification of putative pheromone receptors. Previous reports that examined sexual dimorphism in the antennal lobe of Hawaiian *Drosophila* species identified several prominent lateral glomeruli that are larger in male than female flies.[61] Both DL3 and DA1 are considerably larger in male Hawaiian species than females. The same analysis in *Drosophila melanogaster* indicates that compared to the female, the male DA1 and VA1m+l are 62% and 33% larger, respectively, while DL3 and VA1d are isomorphic in both sexes.[61] These glomeruli receive input from OSNs expressing *Or67d* (DA1) and *Or47b* (VA1m+l),[29,30] both of which are housed in trichoid sensilla.[29] The basis for this size increase in males is unknown, but earlier investigators noticed that there is also a sexual dimorphism in sensilla number.[33,36] Males have more trichoid sensilla and fewer basiconic sensilla than females.[33,36] Finally, neurons expressing *fruitless*, the master transcriptional regulator of sex-specific development and behavior project to these large lateral, sexually dimorphic glomeruli (Fig. 4, pink hatched glomeruli).[62,69] Thus the hypothesis that male antennae are more sensitive to pheromones, as has been shown for a large number of other insects and that this sensitivity is mediated by specialized pheromone-sensing OSNs housed in trichoid sensilla is well supported by the available data.

Concluding Remarks

The advanced state of knowledge concerning gene expression and synaptic organization of the early olfactory system of the fly makes this a compelling system to address questions in odor coding. For instance, it is not yet clear in any species how and where odor concentration is encoded; how the brain solves odor mixture problems, by far the most likely physiological stimulus an animal will encounter; and how discrimination between perceptually similar odors is achieved.[70] Functional calcium imaging[71-73] and electrophysiology[74,75] will be important tools in future research that seeks to answer these important questions at the cellular level. Finally, little is known about how the olfactory system processes odors to produce stereotyped behavioral outputs. The small size, genetic manipulability and availability of robust olfactory behavior paradigms for *Drosophila* olfaction strengthen the role of this little insect as a powerful genetic model system for the foreseeable future.

References

1. Roskies A, Friedman GC, O'Leary DD. Mechanisms and molecules controlling the development of retinal maps. Perspect Dev Neurobiol 1995; 3(1):63-75.
2. Schieber MH. Constraints on somatotopic organization in the primary motor cortex. J Neurophysiol 2001; 86(5):2125-2143.
3. Frostig RD. Functional organization and plasticity in the adult rat barrel cortex: moving out-of-the-box. Curr Opin Neurobiol 2006; 16(4):445-450.
4. Shamma SA. Topographic organization is essential for pitch perception. Proc Natl Acad Sci USA 2004; 101(5):1114-1115.
5. Rubsamen R. Postnatal development of central auditory frequency maps. J Comp Physiol [A] 1992; 170(2):129-143.
6. Dethier VG. The Hungry Fly: A Physiological Study of the Behavior Associated with Feeding. Cambridge: Harvard University Press, 1976.
7. Arora K, Rodrigues V, Joshi S et al. A gene affecting the specificity of the chemosensory neurons of Drosophila. Nature 1987; 330(6143):62-63.
8. Zhang Y, Hoon MA, Chandrashekar J et al. Coding of sweet, bitter and umami tastes: different receptor cells sharing similar signaling pathways. Cell 2003; 112(3):293-301.
9. Marella S, Fischler W, Kong P et al. Imaging taste responses in the fly brain reveals a functional map of taste category and behavior. Neuron 2006; 49(2):285-295.
10. Wang Z, Singhvi A, Kong P et al. Taste representations in the Drosophila brain. Cell 2004; 117(7):981-991.
11. Thorne N, Chromey C, Bray S et al. Taste perception and coding in Drosophila. Curr Biol 2004; 14(12):1065-1079.
12. Jones LM, Fontanini A, Katz DB. Gustatory processing: a dynamic systems approach. Curr Opin Neurobiol 2006; 16(4):420-428.
13. Glendinning JI, Davis A, Rai M. Temporal coding mediates discrimination of "bitter" taste stimuli by an insect. J Neurosci 2006; 26(35):8900-8908.
14. Firestein S. How the olfactory system makes sense of scents. Nature 2001; 413(6852):211-218.
15. Araneda RC, Kini AD, Firestein S. The molecular receptive range of an odorant receptor. Nat Neurosci 2000; 3(12):1248-1255.
16. Malnic B, Hirono J, Sato T et al. Combinatorial receptor codes for odors. Cell 1999; 96(5):713-723.
17. Hallem EA, Ho MG, Carlson JR. The molecular basis of odor coding in the Drosophila antenna. Cell 2004; 117(7):965-979.
18. Katada S, Hirokawa T, Oka Y et al. Structural basis for a broad but selective ligand spectrum of a mouse olfactory receptor: mapping the odorant-binding site. J Neurosci 2005; 25(7):1806-1815.
19. Hildebrand JG, Shepherd GM. Mechanisms of olfactory discrimination: converging evidence for common principles across phyla. Annu Rev Neurosci 1997; 20:595-631.

20. Strausfeld NJ, Hildebrand JG. Olfactory systems: common design, uncommon origins? Curr Opin Neurobiol 1999; 9(5):634-639.
21. Gao Q, Yuan B, Chess A. Convergent projections of Drosophila olfactory neurons to specific glomeruli in the antennal lobe. Nat Neurosci 2000; 3(8):780-785.
22. Mombaerts P, Wang F, Dulac C et al. Visualizing an olfactory sensory map. Cell 1996; 87(4):675-686.
23. Ressler KJ, Sullivan SL, Buck LB. Information coding in the olfactory system: evidence for a stereotyped and highly organized epitope map in the olfactory bulb. Cell 1994; 79(7):1245-1255.
24. Vassar R, Chao SK, Sitcheran R et al. Topographic organization of sensory projections to the olfactory bulb. Cell 1994; 79(6):981-991.
25. Vosshall LB, Wong AM, Axel R. An olfactory sensory map in the fly brain. Cell 2000; 102:147-159.
26. Uchida N, Takahashi YK, Tanifuji M et al. Odor maps in the mammalian olfactory bulb: domain organization and odorant structural features. Nat Neurosci 2000; 3(10):1035-1043.
27. Mori K, Nagao H, Yoshihara Y. The olfactory bulb: coding and processing of odor molecule information. Science 1999; 286(5440):711-715.
28. Friedrich RW, Korsching SI. Combinatorial and chemotopic odorant coding in the zebrafish olfactory bulb visualized by optical imaging. Neuron 1997; 18(5):737-752.
29. Couto A, Alenius M, Dickson BJ. Molecular, anatomical and functional organization of the Drosophila olfactory system. Curr Biol 2005; 15(17):1535-1547.
30. Fishilevich E, Vosshall LB. Genetic and functional subdivision of the Drosophila antennal lobe. Curr Biol 2005; 15(17):1548-1553.
31. Galizia CG, Sachse S, Rappert A et al. The glomerular code for odor representation is species specific in the honeybee Apis mellifera. Nat Neurosci 1999; 2(5):473-478.
32. Hallem EA, Carlson JR. Coding of odors by a receptor repertoire. Cell 2006; 125(1):143-160.
33. Stocker RF. The organization of the chemosensory system in Drosophila melanogaster: a review. Cell Tissue Res 1994; 275(1):3-26.
34. Clyne P, Grant A, O'Connell R et al. Odorant response of individual sensilla on the Drosophila antenna. Invert Neurosci 1997; 3:127-135.
35. Shanbhag SR, Mueller B, Steinbrecht RA. Atlas of olfactory organs of Drosophila melanogaster. 2. Internal organization and cellular architecture of olfactory sensilla. Arthr Struct Dev 2000; 29:211-229.
36. Shanbhag SR, Mueller B, Steinbrecht RA. Atlas of olfactory organs of Drosophila melanogaster. 1. Types, external organization, innervation and distribution of olfactory sensilla. Int J Insect Morphol Embryol 1999; 28(4):377-397.
37. Reddy GV, Gupta B, Ray K et al. Development of the Drosophila olfactory sense organs utilizes cell-cell interactions as well as lineage. Development 1997; 124(3):703-712.
38. Gupta BP, Rodrigues V. Atonal is a proneural gene for a subset of olfactory sense organs in Drosophila. Genes Cells 1997; 2(3):225-233.
39. Sen A, Reddy GV, Rodrigues V. Combinatorial expression of Prospero, Seven-up and Elav identifies progenitor cell types during sense-organ differentiation in the Drosophila antenna. Dev Biol 2003; 254(1):79-92.
40. Goulding SE, zur Lage P, Jarman AP. amos, a proneural gene for Drosophila olfactory sense organs that is regulated by lozenge. Neuron 2000; 25:69-78.
41. Buck L, Axel R. A novel multigene family may encode odorant receptors: a molecular basis for odor recognition. Cell 1991; 65(1):175-187.
42. Vosshall LB, Amrein H, Morozov PS et al. A spatial map of olfactory receptor expression in the Drosophila antenna. Cell 1999; 96(5):725-736.
43. Clyne PJ, Warr CG, Freeman MR et al. A novel family of divergent seven-transmembrane proteins: candidate odorant receptors in Drosophila. Neuron 1999; 22(2):327-338.
44. Gao Q, Chess A. Identification of candidate Drosophila olfactory receptors from genomic DNA sequence. Genomics 1999; 60(1):31-39.
45. Robertson HM, Warr CG, Carlson JR. Molecular evolution of the insect chemoreceptor gene superfamily in Drosophila melanogaster. Proc Natl Acad Sci USA 2003; 100 Suppl 2:14537-14542.
46. Benton R, Sachse S, Michnick SW et al. Atypical membrane topology and heteromeric function of Drosophila odorant receptors in vivo. PLoS Biol 2006; 4(2):e20.
47. Wistrand M, Kall L, Sonnhammer EL. A general model of G protein-coupled receptor sequences and its application to detect remote homologs. Protein Sci 2006; 15(3):509-521.
48. Fishilevich E, Domingos AI, Asahina K et al. Chemotaxis behavior mediated by single larval olfactory neurons in Drosophila. Curr Biol 2005; 15(23):2086-2096.
49. Kreher SA, Kwon JY, Carlson JR. The molecular basis of odor coding in the Drosophila larva. Neuron 2005; 46:445-456.

50. Ressler KJ, Sullivan SL, Buck LB. A zonal organization of odorant receptor gene expression in the olfactory epithelium. Cell 1993; 73(3):597-609.

51. Vassar R, Ngai J, Axel R. Spatial segregation of odorant receptor expression in the mammalian olfactory epithelium. Cell 1993; 74(2):309-318.

52. Bhalerao S, Sen A, Stocker R et al. Olfactory neurons expressing identified receptor genes project to subsets of glomeruli within the antennal lobe of Drosophila melanogaster. J Neurobiol 2003; 54(4):577-592.

53. Serizawa S, Miyamichi K, Nakatani H et al. Negative feedback regulation ensures the one receptor-one olfactory neuron rule in mouse. Science 2003; 302(5653):2088-2094.

54. Larsson MC, Domingos AI, Jones WD et al. Or83b encodes a broadly expressed odorant receptor essential for Drosophila olfaction. Neuron 2004; 43:703-714.

55. Neuhaus EM, Gisselmann G, Zhang W et al. Odorant receptor heterodimerization in the olfactory system of Drosophila melanogaster. Nat Neurosci 2004; 8:15-17.

56. Goldman AL, Van der Goes van Naters W, Lessing D et al. Coexpression of two functional odor receptors in one neuron. Neuron 2005; 45(5):661-666.

57. de Bruyne M, Clyne PJ, Carlson JR. Odor coding in a model olfactory organ: the Drosophila maxillary palp. J Neurosci 1999; 19(11):4520-4532.

58. de Bruyne M, Foster K, Carlson JR. Odor coding in the Drosophila antenna. Neuron 2001; 30(2):537-552.

59. Yao CA, Ignell R, Carlson JR. Chemosensory coding by neurons in the coeloconic sensilla of the Drosophila antenna. J Neurosci 2005; 25(37):8359-8367.

60. Ha TS, Smith DP. A pheromone receptor mediates 11-cis-vaccenyl acetate-induced responses in Drosophila. J Neurosci 2006; 26(34):8727-8733.

61. Kondoh Y, Kaneshiro KY, Kimura K et al. Evolution of sexual dimorphism in the olfactory brain of Hawaiian Drosophila. Proc R Soc Lond B 2003; 270(1519):1005-1013.

62. Manoli DS, Foss M, Villella A et al. Male-specific fruitless specifies the neural substrates of Drosophila courtship behaviour. Nature 2005; 436:395-400.

63. Stockinger P, Kvitsiani D, Rotkopf S et al. Neural circuitry that governs Drosophila male courtship behavior. Cell 2005; 121(5):795-807.

64. Dobritsa AA, van der Goes van Naters W, Warr CG et al. Integrating the molecular and cellular basis of odor coding in the Drosophila antenna. Neuron 2003; 37(5):827-841.

65. Suh GS, Wong AM, Hergarden AC et al. A single population of olfactory sensory neurons mediates an innate avoidance behaviour in Drosophila. Nature 2004; 431(7010):854-859.

66. Scott K, Brady R, Jr., Cravchik A et al. A chemosensory gene family encoding candidate gustatory and olfactory receptors in Drosophila. Cell 2001; 104(5):661-673.

67. Jones WD, Cayirlioglu P, Kadow IG et al. Two chemosensory receptors together mediate carbon dioxide detection in Drosophila. Nature 2007; 445:86-90.

68. Laissue PP, Reiter C, Hiesinger PR et al. Three-dimensional reconstruction of the antennal lobe in Drosophila melanogaster. J Comp Neurol 1999; 405(4):543-552.

69. Sachse S, Galizia CG. Role of inhibition for temporal and spatial odor representation in olfactory output neurons: A calcium imaging study. J Neurophysiol 2002; 87:1106-1117.

70. Wilson RI, Mainen ZF. Early events in olfactory processing. Annu Rev Neurosci 2006; 29:163-201.

71. Fiala A, Spall T, Diegelmann S et al. Genetically expressed cameleon in Drosophila melanogaster is used to visualize olfactory information in projection neurons. Curr Biol 2002; 12(21):1877-1884.

72. Ng M, Roorda RD, Lima SQ et al. Transmission of olfactory information between three populations of neurons in the antennal lobe of the fly. Neuron 2002; 36(3):463-474.

73. Wang JW, Wong AM, Flores J et al. Two-photon calcium imaging reveals an odor-evoked map of activity in the fly brain. Cell 2003; 112(2):271-282.

74. Wilson RI, Laurent G. Role of GABAergic inhibition in shaping odor-evoked spatiotemporal patterns in the Drosophila antennal lobe. J Neurosci 2005; 25(40):9069-9079.

75. Wilson RI, Turner GC, Laurent G. Transformation of olfactory representations in the Drosophila antennal lobe. Science 2004; 303(5656):366-370.

CHAPTER 8

Optic Lobe Development

Karl-Friedrich Fischbach* and Peter Robin Hiesinger

Abstract

The optic lobes comprise approximately half of the fly's brain. In four major synaptic ganglia, or neuropils, the visual input from the compound eyes is received and processed for higher order visual functions like motion detection and color vision. A common characteristic of vertebrate and invertebrate visual systems is the point-to-point mapping of the visual world to synaptic layers in the brain, referred to as visuotopy. Vision requires the parallel extraction of numerous parameters in a visuotopic manner. Consequently, the optic neuropils are arranged in columns and perpendicularly oriented synaptic layers that allow for the selective establishment of synapses between columnar neurons. How this exquisite synaptic specificity is established during approximately 100 hours of brain development is still poorly understood. However, the optic lobe contains one of the best characterized brain structures in any organism—both anatomically and developmentally. Moreover, numerous molecules and their function illuminate some of the basic mechanisms involved in brain wiring. The emerging picture is that the development of the visual system of *Drosophila* is (epi-)genetically hard-wired; it supplies the emerging fly with vision without requiring neuronal activity for fine tuning of neuronal connectivity. Elucidating the genetic and cellular principles by which gene activity directs the assembly of the optic lobe is therefore a fascinating task and the focus of this chapter.

Introduction

Several comprehensive works cover the description of early events during optic lobe development in *Drosophila*,[1-3] whereas most recent reviews focus on the molecules and mechanisms during the establishment of synaptic connectivity in the visual system.[4-6] The present chapter focuses on optic lobe development from the viewpoint of neurogenetics: How can a surprisingly low number of genes encode the wiring of a complicated brain structure? An answer must encompass all levels of the developmental program, from cellular differentiation and movement to the molecules and mechanisms that provide meaningful synapse formation signals. In particular, we will focus on the events and mechanisms that lead to the recognition of synaptic partners. What is the mechanism of such recognition events? What are the molecular players at the level of the cell surface during recognition events and what are the mechanisms for their precise, dynamically regulated expression pattern? And, finally, how plastic is this program, i.e., to what extent is the final synaptic wiring pattern determined by the genetic program?

Recognition of different cell types is not confined to the nervous system and is a general requirement in the development of multicellular organisms. Without cell recognition, recruitment of cells into developing tissues would be impossible. Recognition between different cell types is especially demanding in the nervous system where neurons have to synapse with specific partners, often thousands of cell body diameters apart. Due to their regular, columnar and layered organization visual

*Corresponding Author: Karl-Friedrich Fischbach—Department of Neurobiology,
Albert-Ludwigs-University of Freiburg, Schaenzlestr.1, D-79104 Freiburg, Germany.
Email: kff@uni-freiburg.de

Brain Development in Drosophila melanogaster, edited by Gerhard M. Technau.
©2008 Landes Bioscience and Springer Science+Business Media.

systems are well suited to investigate the genetic determination and developmental rules that underlie the establishment of neuronal connectivity. The repetitive organization of about 750 visual units or columns on each side of the fly's head allow the detection of minor disturbances. The visual system of *Drosophila* has the further advantage that an exceptionally powerful toolbox can be applied to genetically dissect the developmental programs.

The Adult Visual System Is Organized into Parallel Visuotoptic Functional Pathways

The adult optic lobes of coleoptera, lepidoptera and diptera[7,8] are subdivided into four neuropils, the lamina, medulla, lobula and lobula plate (Figs. 1A, 2A). Photoreceptor projections from the eye directly innervate the first two neuropils, lamina and medulla. In *Drosophila*, each single eye, or ommatidium, of the compound eye contains eight different photoreceptor cell types. Their light-sensing protrusion, the rhabdomeres, receive light along seven different optical axes underneath a single lens. The outer 6 rhabdomeres are formed by retinula cells R1-6; the inner rhabdomere comprises distally R7 and proximally R8. In all ommatidia, except those of the dorsal rim, the inner rhabdomeres are much thinner than the outer ones. Functionally, the outer photoreceptors are responsible for spatial vision, whereas the inner photoreceptors convey color vision.

Three types of ommatidia can be distinguished[9] according to the rhodopsin (Rh) content of the inner retinula cells R7 and R8: 30% of ommatidia are of the pale subtype, where R7 contains the UV-sensitive Rh3 and R8 the blue-sensitive Rh5, while the remaining 70% are of the yellow subtype and contain UV-sensitive Rh4 in R7 and green-sensitive Rh6 in R8. Both types are randomly distributed due to the stochastic expression pattern of the transcription factor and Dioxin receptor homolog *spineless* in R7 cells. The expression of Spineless in R7 cells specifies it as a Rh4 cell. R7 then dictates the fate of the R8 cell to also assume the yellow subtype. In the absence of *spineless* or in *spineless* mutants, all R7 and most R8 cells adopt the pale (Rh5) fate, whereas overexpression of *spineless* is sufficient to induce the yellow R7 fate.[10] The molecular mechanism that determines the stochastic expression of Spineless as well as the functional significance of the random pale/yellow ommatidia distribution are currently unknown.

In addition to these two major ommatidial types there is a dorsal rim area of the compound eyes[9,11] which is specialized for the detection of polarized light. Here R7 and R8 rhabdomeres have larger diameters and both express the UV-sensitive Rh3. As the microvilli of both cell types are perpendicularly oriented with respect to each other, this allows the evaluation of the vector of

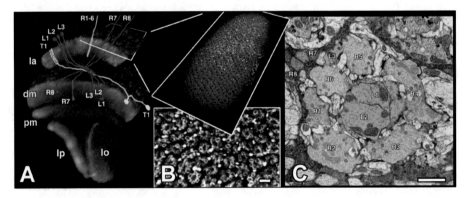

Figure 1. The Drosophila optic lobe. A) Volume rendered optic lobe neuropils based on synaptic staining (n-Syb). Selected characterized cell types are depicted based on Golgi studies.[18] la, lamina; dm, distal medulla; pm, proximal medulla; lp, lobula plate; lo, lobula. B) The primary visual map. Lamina cross-sections of confocal images based on a photoreceptor-specific antibody staining. Scale bar 5μm. C) EM micrograph of a single unit (cartridge) of the visual map in the lamina. Color code as in A. Scale bar 1μm.

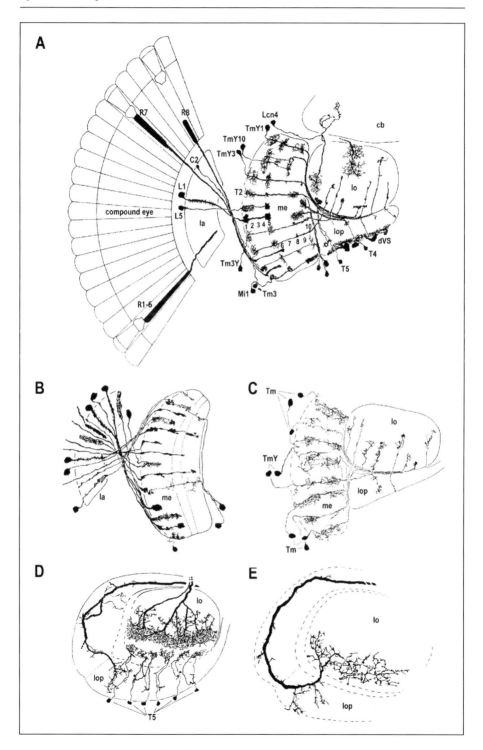

Figure 2, legend viewed on following page.

Figure 2, viewed on previous page. Golgi Gestalten of neurons in wild type and mutant optic lobes. A) Composite scheme of the left compound eye and optic lobe with camera lucida drawings of Golgi impregnated neurons of wild type flies selected to illustrate the layering of the medulla neuropil, e.g., L1, L5, Mi1, Tm3, Tm3Y, T2, TmY3, TmY1, but not TmY10 are potential interactors in the distal medulla as their arborizations overlap in layers M1 and M5 (see numbers without prefix). Original camera lucida drawings taken from Fischbach and Dittrich (1989).[18] B, C) Camera lucida drawings of columnar neurons in the optic lobe of the *small optic lobes^{KS58}* mutant display a partial loss of stratification (modified from[126]). D, E) Camera lucida drawings of some examples of neuronal cell types surviving congenital sensory deprivation in completely eyeless *sine oculis*[2] flies. Sprouting of medulla tangentials into the lobula complex can be seen (modified from[91]). la, lamina; me, medulla; lo, lobula; lop, lobula plate; cb, central brain. Naked numbers 1-10 depict medulla layers M1-M10. dVS, dendrites of giant vertical neurons of the lobula plate; all others labels are names of neuronal cell types following the nomenclature of Fischbach and Dittrich (1989).[18]

light polarization rather than wavelength. The homeodomain transcription factor homothorax is both necessary and sufficient for R7/R8 to adopt the polarization-sensitive dorsal rim fate instead of the color-sensitive default state. Homothorax increases rhabdomere size and uncouples R7-R8 communication to allow both cells to express the same opsin rather than different ones as required for color vision. Homothorax expression is induced by the dorsally expressed genes of the *iroquois* complex and the *wingless (wg)* pathway.[12]

The outer photoreceptors responsible for spatial vision terminate in the first optic ganglion, the lamina, whereas the inner photoreceptors responsible for color vision project through the lamina into the second and major optic neuropil, the medulla (Figs. 1,2). It has to be expected that the different types of R7 and R8 retinula cells described above project to specialized target neurons in the optic lobe. In fact, in the locust, the neuronal pathways of the dorsal rim region could be traced via neurons in the dorsal rim of the medulla to the lower unit of the anterior optic tubercle.[13] It is noteworthy, that the decision about the type of opsin occurs in the midpupal stage, after the axons have found their way into the brain and during the period of synapse specification and formation. It is not known whether the opsin decision also influences target choices in the maturing neuropil of *Drosophila*.

The axons of the eight retinula cells per ommatidium project to the adult brain following the neural superposition rule[14-16] which secures that axons from retinula cells obtaining information from the same point in space project into the same cartridge of the lamina or column of the medulla. In larval development, the R1-6 axons of a single ommatidium form a common fascicle with their leading R8 axon and follow it through the larval optic stalk into the larval lamina plexus in a retinotopic fashion. They distribute themselves to six different, neighbouring lamina cartridges and establish a visuotopically correct map only later.[2,17] The R8 and the following R7 axons directly project into the medulla in a correct retino- and visuotopic manner, as discussed in detail in section 4 of this chapter. The six outer R-cell terminals of a single ommatidium are presynaptic to the dendrites of lamina monopolar neurons L1, L2 and L3 in six different lamina cartridges, while the L-cell dendrites receive input from R-cells coming from six different ommatidia. The axons of the lamina monopolar cells L1-5 (only the first three are postsynaptic to R1-6) of a single cartridge project via the first optic chiasm into specific layers of isotopic medulla columns (Figs. 2,3). While a single lamina cartridge receives input from retinula cells with identical optical axes of six neighbouring ommatidia, a medulla column samples such information from 7 ommatidia, transmitted via 5 different direct neuronal channels (L1, L2, L3, R7 and R8).

In summary, while R7 and R8 directly form retinotopic projections in the medulla, R1-R6 undergo axon terminal resorting according to the principle of neural superposition to match the orientation of the optical axes of the adult rhabdomeres (visuotopy). The visuotopic organization is a general feature of all image processing visual systems in invertebrates as well as in vertebrates.

Most of the visual interneurons of *Drosophila* have been described in Golgi studies.[18] They can be classified into many columnar and fewer tangential types, the axons of which are oriented perpendicular to each other. By mere evaluation of the structural features (Fig. 2A) it has been

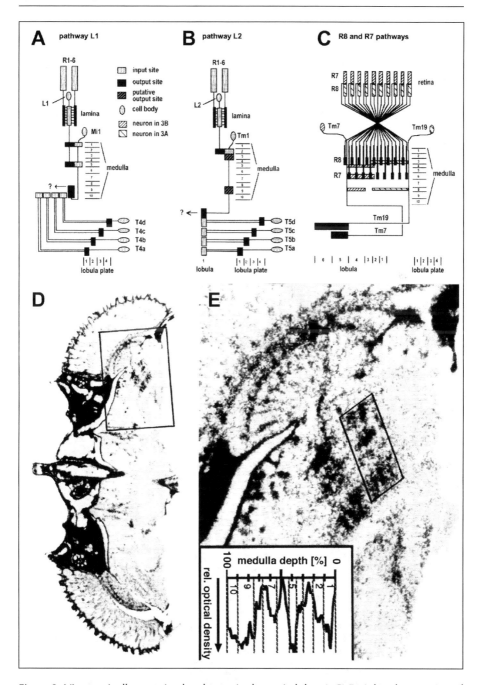

Figure 3. Visuotopically organized pathways in the optic lobe. A-C) Peripheral separation of visuotopically organized functional pathways requires the organization of the optic lobe in columns and layers. Three functional pathways in the optic lobe are shown which are inferred from the relationship of layered arborizations of all known cellular Golgi profiles. Legend continued on following page.

Figure 3, viewed on previous page. For simplicity, at the level of the medulla only typical neuronal types are shown. The L1 and L2 pathways are fed by R1-6 and function in spatial vision,
the R8 and R7 pathways in color vision. D) depicts an ^{3}H-2-deoxyglucose autoradiogram of a
horizontal brain section after unilateral 120 min stimulation in two 15 × 15 degree sectors of
the right visual field. The right optic lobe autoradiogram is enlarged in E. The anterior visual
field window (posterior medulla sector) was stimulated by upward motion, the posterior
visual field window by horizontal progressive motion of the same spatial wavelength (using
a sinusoidally modulated gray scale). In both cases visuotopically situated columnar neurons
of the L1 and L2 pathway layers (A,B) have taken up radioactive deoxyglucose. The density
profile of the medulla sector stimulated by upward motion is shown in the inset. It is obvious
that the R7/R8 pathway layers M3 and M6 are silent under these conditions (modified from
Fischbach et al 1992[22]).

claimed that several, visuotopically organized, parallel visual pathways co-exist[19] (Fig. 3A-C). In
combination with 2-deoxyglucose studies[20] a clear structural separation between the pathways for
motion detection and colour vision could be demonstrated[18-22] (see Fig. 3D,E).

   This neuronal organization of the visual system of *Drosophila* contrasts sharply with the olfactory system, where olfactory receptor cells with the same chemosensory specificity converge in so
called glomeruli of the antennal lobe onto single large interneurons (relay neurons) that project
to the mushroom bodies and the lateral protocerebrum[23,24] (see Chapters by R. Stocker and by
V. Rodrigues and T. Hummel). However, it has recently been pointed out that the output level
of the visual system is also comparable to the olfactory system, as visuotopically organized lobula
output neurons of the same type converge in so-called optic glomeruli, where they synapse onto
large projection neurons[25,26] (Fig. 4). It is therefore tempting to suggest that the visuotopic, parallel
pathway organization is an evolutionary added feature of the visual system.

   What is known about the cellular and molecular mechanisms that enable the visuotopic and
pathway-specific wiring in the optic lobe? We will first review data related to the dependence
of visual neuropil development on retinal innervation and will consider some of the functions
of known cellular and molecular factors involved in axonal pathfinding, target recognition and
synaptogenesis.

Lamina Development

Retinal Innervation: Axon Outgrowth and Interdependence with Optic Lobe Development

   Axon outgrowth from the retina occurs in a developmental wave following the wave of cellular
differentiation in the eye disc. The first (pioneer) axons grow out from R8, followed by R2&R5,
R3&R4, then R1&R6 and R7 follow last.[27] The retinal axons project through the tubular optic
stalk that consists of a monolayer of surface glia and forms before axon ingrowth under the control the
focal adhesion kinase Fak56D.[28] The larval photoreceptor organ, the Bolwig's organ, is dispensable
for adult wild-type photoreceptor axons to project normally and is thus not an essential pioneer of
axonal navigation to the lamina. Bolwig's organ later transforms into the four photoreceptors of an
extra-retinal posterior "eyelet", the so-called "Hofbauer-Buchner eyelet",[29] which is involved in the
generation of circadian rhythm.[30] The best characterized signal transduction pathway required for
photoreceptor growth cone guidance includes the Insulin receptor on the cell surface[31] and intracel-
lularly *dreadlocks* (*dock*, a SH2/SH3 adaptor protein), *pak* (p21 activated protein kinase), *trio* (a
Rho family guanine exchange factor that activates Rac), *misshapen* (a Ste20-like serine/threonine
kinase) and *bifocal* (a putative cytoskeletal regulator).[32-37] These molecular components have been
proposed to constitute a signal transduction cascade from the cell surface to the actin cytoskeleton.
Targeting choices of the different photoreceptor subtypes and the upstream guidance receptors
are described in more detail below.

   While maintainance of the fly's retina requires that retinal axons connect to the optic lobe,[25]
it is well established that retinae develop quite normally in ectopic positions without connections
to the brain, either achieved by transplantation[38] or by ectopic expression of eyeless.[39] Also the

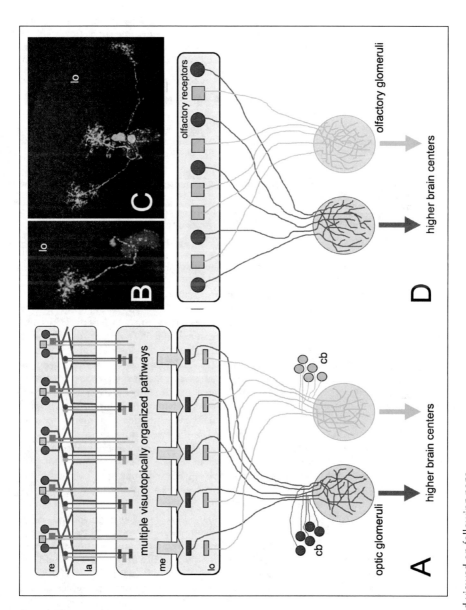

Figure 4. Legend viewed on following page.

Figure 4, viewed on previous page. Comparing wiring principles of the olfactory and the visual system. A) Schematic view of the visual system. Visuotopy is maintained up to the lobula complex (lobula plate has been omitted for simplicity). Different sets of lobula columnar neurons project to specific optic glomeruli, where they terminate in a nonvisuotopic manner. B,C) GFP marked neurons resulting from MARCM using the *irreC/rst*-specific Gal4 driver NP2044. Background staining with an IrreC/Rst-specific antibody. B) The terminals of a single LC12 neuron branch throughout its glomerulus. C) A clone of three such LC12 neurons subserving different parts of the visual field are shown. D) Schematic view of the organization of the olfactory system. Here all olfactory receptor cells of the same kind directly project to the same glomerulus. re, retina; la, lamina; me, medulla; lo, lobula; cb, cell bodies.

unconnected phenotype of the *disconnected* mutant, in which the retinula cell axons of the compound eye do not connect to the brain, demonstrates that retina development, which proceeds normally, is autonomous.[40] This does not hold for the optic lobe, the development of which strongly depends on retinal innervation (Fig. 2D,E). It was already demonstrated by Power in 1943 and confirmed by Hinke in 1961 that optic lobe volume strongly correlates with the facet number of the compound eye.[41,42] In his volumetric studies Power found that eyeless flies do not develop a lamina at all and have a drastically reduced medulla and lobula complex (about 80% and 60% reduction respectively).

Optic lobe interneurons are the progeny of two groups of progenitor cells, arranged in the outer and inner optic anlagen. The lamina (together with the distal part of the medulla, see below) arise from the outer optic anlage.[43] The strong correlation of lamina size with the number of ommatidia is the direct consequence of an inductive influence of ingrowing retinula (R) cell axons on neurogenesis of lamina neurons[44,45] and lamina glia.[46] Photoreceptor innervation thus triggers the final cell-cycle of lamina precursor cells. Hedgehog, that is released from R-cell axons, induces the generation of lamina monopolar neurons from lamina precursor cells which—in the absence of Hedgehog—are arrested in the G1 phase.[47-49] Hedgehog transport in photoreceptors has recently been shown to depend on the competition between targeting signals of the Hedgehog N- and C-termini. After Hedgehog cleavage, the N-terminal domain is targeted to the retina, while the C-terminal domain is responsible for Hedgehog transport along the axon.[50] Together with Hedgehog, the epidermal growth factor receptor (EGFR) ligand Spitz is transported down the photoreceptor axons. The postsynaptic precursor cells express EGFR and are thus initiated to assemble the postsynaptic cell complement for the lamina cartridge.[47] By the concerted action of Hedgehog and Spitz, the number of presynaptic neurons determines the size of the postsynaptic neuronal population. The five lamina cell types L1-L5 are thereby specified. As young retinal ommatidia are added anteriorly, this also implies that the lamina grows from posterior to anterior. Lamina precursor cells as well as glia cells require the transcription factor Glia cells missing (*gcm*) and Glia cells missing 2 (*gcm2*), that were previously thought to be exclusively required for glial cell fate determination.[51] Of further importance on the side of the lamina precursor cells is the gene product of *dally*. In *dally* loss-of-function mutants the lamina precursors do not perform the second division that is triggered by ingrowing retinal fibres.[52] Dally is a heparan sulfate proteoglycan attached to the membrane via a GPI-anchor and able to modulate Hedgehog signaling.[53]

The dependence of lamina differentiation upon the ingrowth of retinal fibres provides a straight-forward programming of retinotopic projections along the anterior-posterior axis. As a wave of differentiation (visible as the so-called morphogenetic furrow) sweeps along the eye-imaginal disc from posterior to anterior during the late larval and early pupal stage, the new ommatidial axon bundles leave the eye imaginal disc anteriorly and accordingly induce lamina development also at its anterior margin.[27,54] Maturation of the eye imaginal disc and the lamina therefore occurs in parallel from posterior to anterior. Apoptosis of excess cells concludes the wave of development in the lamina. In vertebrates, Eph receptor tyrosine kinases have critical roles in retinotopic map formation. *Drosophila* contains only one Eph gene, which has indeed been implicated in the targeting of retinotopic projections, although the precise cellular requirement and mechanism are less clear.[55]

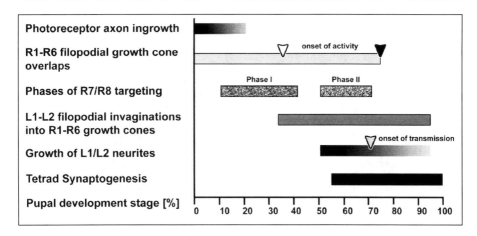

Figure 5. Timeline of morphogenetic events during pupal optic lobe wiring. Depicted is the temporal succession of different phases of photoreceptor and lamina monopolar cell (L1/L2) growth, incorporating data from different fly species. Innervation of the anterior lamina by photoreceptors axons is complete by 20% of pupal development. Transient filopodial-growth cone invaginations and overlaps amongst R1-R6 growth cones can be observed up to 75% of pupal development. The arrowheads show the approximate onset of R1-R6 responses recorded using sharp electrodes in the blowfly *Calliphora* (open arrowhead)[127] or whole-cell recordings (filled arrowhead) from dissociated ommatidia in *Drosophila*.[128] In the first half of pupal development R1-R6 terminals are resorted according to the neural superposition rule.[2,17] Two phases of R7/R8 target layer selection have been distinguished in the medulla.[98] Growth of L1/L2 neurites and filopodial growth cone invaginations from at least one L1/L2 axon into R1-R6 growth cones can be observed through most of the second half of pupation. The grey arrowhead indicates the approximate onset of synaptic transmission to L1/L2 based on *Calliphora* data.[127] Synaptogenesis takes place in the second half of pupal development and culminates in the formation of tetrads which unite elements of four different cell types at a single synapse.[2] Modified from I. A. Meinertzhagen et al (2000).[129]

No such helpful temporal gradient does exist when the establishment of retinotopy along the dorso-ventral axes is considered. How is it secured that dorsal retinula axons project into the dorsal lamina and ventral retinula axons project into the ventral lamina? By the use of eye mutants with reduced facet number, it was demonstrated that navigation of ommatidial bundles is independent of each other: Single bundles navigate more or less correctly in the absence of neighbouring one. Genetically wild type axons are even able to innervate their correct brain region, when surrounding fibres are misprojecting due to the glass genotype.[56] Which cues are these axons using for their navigation?

DWnt4, a *Drosophila* member of the Wnt family of secreted glycoproteins, is specifically expressed in the ventral half of the developing lamina in the third instar larval stage.[57] In the absence of DWnt4, ventral retinal axons misproject to the dorsal lamina and can be redirected towards an ectopic source of DWnt4. Wnt glycoproteins are known to activate via Frizzled (Fz) receptors canonical (ß-catenin dependent) as well as noncanonical (ß-catenin independent) signaling pathways. Ventral retinula cells missing the Dfrizzled2 (Dfz2) receptor or the directly interacting Dishevelled protein often misroute their axons dorsally and it could be shown that interference with noncanonical but not with canonical signaling affects axon targeting along the dorso-ventral axis. These results suggest that secreted DWnt4 from the ventral lamina acts as an attractant for retinal axons that express Dfz2. In dorsal retinula cells the expression of the genes of the *iroquois* complex seem to attenuate the competence of Dfz2 to respond to DWnt4.[57]

Stop and Go at The Marginal Glia

In the larva, the lamina neuropil (called lamina plexus at this stage) contains the R1-6 terminals and is sandwiched between layers of glial cells. Distally of the R1-6 terminals, the epithelial glial cells are situated and proximally the lamina marginal glial cells. They separate the R1-6 terminals from the layer of medulla glia. Several lines of evidence suggest that the lamina marginal glial cells represent an intermediate target for R1-6 growth cones and cause them to stop at this point. In nonstop mutants[58,59] glial cell development is disrupted and the axons of R1-6 do not terminate in the lamina, but project down into the medulla. Nonstop is a ubiquitin-specific protease that is required in glia cells. Similarly, the absence of marginal glia in clones mutant for *Medea*, which codes for a DPP signal transducer, results in R1-6 axon projection defects.[60]

Contacting glial cells as intermediate targets may be the price retinula cells have to pay for regulating the neurogenesis of their postsynaptic partners. These still have to differentiate and it is not before the second half of pupal development that synapses are being formed[2,61,62] (Fig. 5).

Neither the molecular nature of the stop signal emitted by marginal glial cells nor the receptor in R-cells are currently known. However, it was shown that the absence of the receptor tyrosine phosphatase PTP69D in photoreceptors sometimes leads to their projection into the medulla.[63] As PTP69D is also required for the correct targeting of R7 to layer M6 of the medulla (in its absence R7 terminates in M3 like R8) it has been suggested that PTP69D plays a permissive role in R1-6 and R7 axonal targeting by helping to defasciculate from the leading R8 axon.[64]

After having stopped at the marginal glia, R1-6 growth cones are hanging around for quite a while. Apparently the reception of nitric oxide (NO), which is produced by lamina cells, is required for these growth cones not to project further down into the medulla.[65] Furthermore, Brakeless, a nuclear protein is needed in retinula cells to stop their axons at the marginal glia.[66,67] Interestingly, Brakeless acts as a transcriptional repressor of the *runt* pair rule gene, which encodes the Runt transcription factor required for R7 and R8 axonal projections into the medulla. If repression of *runt* by Brakeless is abolished in R2 and R5 cells only, this is sufficient to induce the projection of all six outer R-cells into the medulla.[68] This fact clearly indicates the existence of interactions between the R-cell terminals in larval development. As R2 and R5 are determined directly after the R8-cell, their axons are the first to follow the R8 axon. When the first three axons of an ommatidial bundle project into the medulla, the trailing axons might be forced to follow due to fasciculative forces. During the pupal stage, afferent-afferent interactions also seem to play an important role in the sprouting of the outer R-cell terminals to their correct visuotopic cartridges.[2,17,69]

Neural Superposition: Correcting the Initial Retinotopic Projections in the Lamina

Initially, in the larvae, all outer R-cell axons from a single ommatidium form a single fascicle. They terminate together, sandwiched between the epithelial and marginal glia in the lamina plexus, retaining their spatial relationship in the ommatidium. A column of 5 lamina monopolar neurons is induced by the incoming photoreceptors distally. Lamina monopolar axons fasciculate with the R7/8 axons of the corresponding ommatidium and project towards the medulla. Due to the axonal ingrowth from new ommatidia and the corresponding recruitment of lamina neurons and glia along the posterior—anterior axes, a precise retinotopic map is established. However, the retinotopic map is of little use for R1-R6 in the lamina, as the R1-R6 from a single ommatidium look at different points in visual space. In order to obtain a visuotopic map from here, R-cell axons have to be resorted so that axons coming from retinula cells looking at the same point in space in the adult are united in a single cartridge. This process takes place in the first half of pupal development[2,17] (see Figs. 5,6). It is interesting to note that the extensive resorting and hence rewiring of photoreceptor terminals in the lamina is a peculiarity solely made necessary by the fact that *Drosophila* ommatidia, like all Diptera, contain a split or open rhabdom system; the rhabdomeres receive light from different points in space under the same lens. A single secreted protein, Spacemaker, is necessary and sufficient for the formation of an open system.[70]

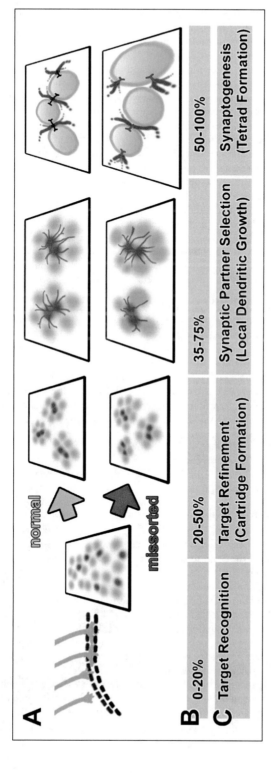

Figure 6. The Development of the Drosophila Visual Map. Time series of developmental steps normally leading to the formation of visuotopically correct synapses. A) R1-R6 growth cones initially stop at the marginal glia. Sorting of photoreceptor terminals into cartridges that map neighboring points in space occurs during the first half of pupal development. The second half is characterized by synapse formation between synaptic partners that were prespecified during cartridge formation. A normal number of synapses forms in photoreceptor terminals independent of synaptic partner accuracy. Green, photoreceptor terminals; red, postsynaptic lamina monopolar cells. B) Time scale. C) Naming of developmental steps. Adapted from Hiesinger et al 2006[71].

By visualizing projections from single ommatidia labeled with DiI and by deleting subsets of retinula cells, it was demonstrated that interactions among the R-cell population itself regulate cartridge selection.[17] First it was shown that remaining R-cell terminals in mutants for *phyllopod* (R1, R6 and R7 are transformed into cone cells), *lozenge*[sprite] (transforms R3 and R4 into R7 cells) and *seven-up* (transforms R3 and R4 and in addition R1 and R6 into R7) are still able to defasciculate and to initiate their search for a lamina target. Therefore, this basic behavior seems to be independent of other R-terminals in the bundle. However, when R1 and R6 were absent, the final projections of the remaining R3 and R4 terminals were invariably correct, while those of R2 and R5 sometimes showed defects. R1 and R6 are therefore not required for the correct projections of R3 and R4, but do influence R2 and R5 targeting. In *lozenge*[sprite], absence of R3 and R4 leads to highly aberrant targeting of the remaining R-cell axons (R1, R2, R5, R6). In the *seven-up* mutant, where in addition R1 and R6 are missing, the remaining R2 and R5 are always making targeting errors.[17] In conclusion these results indicate a specific interaction between R-cell axons with regard to their final projections in the lamina.

Mutations in many genes have been identified in large screens using the eyFLP method[64] that affect this photoreceptor terminal resorting and thus lead to cartridges with too few or too many R-cell terminals.[71] The list contains several guidance receptors and cell adhesion molecules, including DLar (a receptor tyrosine phosphatase), DN-Cadherin (a classical cadherin) and Flamingo (a protocadherin).[72-74] For N-Cadherin mediation of attractive interaction between photoreceptor axons during visual map formation has been demonstrated.[75] All of these are also required for the targeting of R7/R8 in the medulla, as discussed in more detail below.

Guidance cues like the above-mentioned cell adhesion molecules must be accurately spatiotemporally regulated and localized in order to provide meaningful synapse formation signals. Vesicle trafficking has been implicated in the localization of cell adhesion molecules in photoreceptors mutant for neuronal synaptobrevin, which encodes a vesicle protein critically required for vesicle fusion.[76] More recently, loss of a vesicle-associated protein, the exocyst component Sec15, has been shown to cause specific cartridge sorting and R7/R8 projection defects (Fig. 7). Importantly, photoreceptors mutant for *sec15* display mislocalization phenotypes for a specific subset of guidance molecules, including DLar.[77] Which intracellular compartments are responsible for the dynamic and precise trafficking and localization of guidance receptors is unknown.

Synapse Formation in the Lamina Is Activity-Independent and Synapse Number Is Presynaptically Determined

In vertebrates the refinement of retinotopic maps in the visual system is strongly affected by electric neuronal activity and by competition between presynaptic terminals.[78,79] Although visual deprivation in early adulthood does reduce synapse number in the visual system of *Drosophila*,[80] neuronal activity is not required for synaptic partner selection, synapse formation or refinement of synapse numbers in pupal photoreceptors. The emerging fly is thus provided with a prespecified, functional visual system that has been built by activity-independent mechanisms.[71] The argument is based on the evaluation of the brain structure of mutants with defects in the generation of electrical potentials (*norpA*[P24]: phospholipase C, required for phototransduction[81] and *trp*[343]; *trpl*[302]: Ca²⁺ channels required for evoked and spontaneous electrical potentials), or with defects in the conduction of electrical potentials (*para*[ts1]: sodium channel), or with defects in the release of neurotransmitter (*hdcjk910*, a histidine decarboxylase[82,83]) and *synaptotagmin* (a Ca²⁺-sensor required for neurotransmitter release[84]). Importantly, in spite of the absence of spontaneous or evoked electrical activity, cartridge sorting according to the principle of neural superposition as well as the formation of the correct number of synapses in each cartridge are normal.[71] Per R-cell terminal about 50 evenly spaced synapses are formed.[85,86]

Synapse number is not only independent of electrical activity, but also independent from hypo- or hyperinnervation of a single cartridge by R-cell terminals (Fig. 6). Synapse constancy per R-cell terminal was first suggested for house flies[87] and recently shown for *Drosophila*.[71] In a collection of cartridge missorting mutants, terminals in aberrant cartridges nevertheless form a normal number of synapses with the postsynaptic L1-3 neurons. The number of synapses per R-cell terminal does not correlate with the number of terminals per cartridge, which shows that there is no competition for limited postsynaptic contact provided by L1-3. The presynaptic R-cell terminal is exerting control.[71] Nothing is known about the mechanism that restricts the number of synapses at the presynaptic site.

Medulla and Lobula Complex Development

As compared to the lamina, the neuropils of the medulla and lobula complex are structurally much more complex and house many more neuronal types.[18] Columnar organization is retained and there is a one to one correspondence between lamina cartridges and medulla columns, in spite of the fact that the connecting fibres cross in the outer (first) optic chiasm in the horizontal plane. These fine-grained, isotopic point-to-point connections are also retained between the medulla and the lobula complex through the axon bundles in the inner optic chiasm. However, at the level of the lobula output neurons, the number of repetitive elements is reduced.[26,88,89] While the lamina neuropil is only weakly stratified (e.g., the L4 collaterals are restricted to the proximal lamina layer), stratification of the medulla, lobula and and lobula plate is pronounced (Fig. 2A). Based on profiles of Golgi impregnated neurons, the medulla has been divided into ten different layers (M1-M10), the lobula into six layers (Lo1-Lo6) and the lobula plate into four layers (Lop1-Lop4).[18] Layers M1-M6 constitute the distal medulla and layers M8-10 the proximal medulla. In structural brain mutants like *small optic lobes (sol)*[90] the layering of the neuropil can be severely disturbed (Fig. 2B,C). Both parts of the medulla are separated by the serpentine layer M7, which houses large tangential axons and dendrites of medulla columnar neurons projecting to or from the Cucatti bundle. Columnar neurons of the distal medulla, like lamina monopolar cells, are derived from the outer optic anlage, while columnar neurons of the proximal medulla and the lobula complex derive from the inner optic anlage.[2,43]

In contrast to the lamina, that is completely dependent on retinal innervation, medulla and lobula complex rudiments do exist in completely eyeless flies.[41,91] (Fig. 2D,E). These rudiments are not exclusively built by descendants of the inner optic anlage; they still contain columnar neurons derived from the outer optic anlage[91] and cell loss seems mainly be due to degeneration of differentiated neurons rather than to a lack of proliferation of neuronal precursors, as massive axonal degeneration has been decribed at the level of the inner optic chiam in eyeless *sine oculis* pupae.[92] This indicates that the final division of the precursors of these neurons does not depend on induction by innervation of R7/R8 or of lamina monopolar axons.

It is also very telling that the neuropil rudiments of medulla, lobula and lobula plate are still isotopically connected by columnar neurons in such completely eyeless flies[91] (Fig. 2D). Visuotopy in the wild type optic lobe is therefore not completely induced by the ordered ingrowth of retinula cells. Also layering, at least at the level of the lobula, is partially retained. However, a reliable feature of the optic lobe rudiments of completely eyeless flies is the fusion of the posterior medulla neuropil with the lobula plate. This fusion seems to result from the sprouting of medulla tangentials into the lobula plate[91] (Fig. 2D,E). The relative independence of the deeper layers of optic lobe neuropils from eye development may reflect their intensive invasion by neurons that house their cell bodies in regions of the central brain.[26]

The Importance of Compartment Boundaries

Glial septa define neuronal compartments in the developing central brain as well as in the optic lobe.[93] One such border separates the outer optic anlage and its descendants from the inner optic anlage and its offspring. During development lamina cells are in very close proximity to cells of the lobula cortex. These cell populations never intermingle in wild type flies. The Robo/Slit receptor/ligand system was recently shown to be of importance for the maintenance of the separation of these cell populations. Slit is secreted by lamina glia and repels Robo-positive neurons of the lobula complex.[94] The *egghead (egh)* gene is also involved in the establishment of this compartment border.[95] In the absence of *egh*, some R1-R6 axons project abnormally to the medulla. This

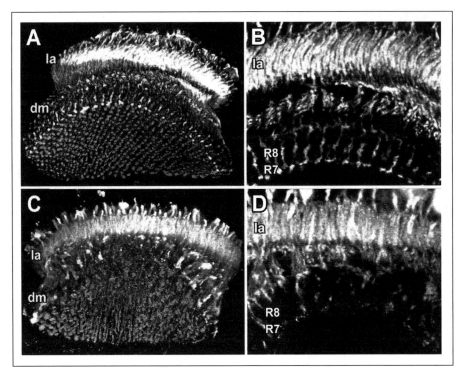

Figure 7. Normal and aberrant photoreceptor projections in the optic lobe. A, C) 3D reconstructions from confocal stacks of photoreceptor projections in newly eclosed flies, viewed from inside the brain. B, D) Projections views of respective brains at higher magnification. A, B) Wild type R1-R6 projections form a dense synaptic layer in the lamina (la). R7/R8 project through the outer chiasm and terminate in separate layers in the medulla (dm, distal medulla). C, D) Mutants defective for correct synaptic partner selection (shown here are photoreceptors mutant for *sec15*) are characterized by a loss of the precise and regular projection pattern in both neuropils (adapted from Mehta et al 2005[77]).

is not due to a loss of *egh* function in the eye or in the neurons and glia of the lamina. Instead, clonal analysis and cell-specific rescue experiments showed that *egh* is required in cells of the lobula complex primordium, which abuts the lamina and medulla in the developing larval brain. In the absence of *egh*, sheath-like glial processes at the boundary region delimiting lamina glia and lobula cortex are in disorder and inappropriate invasion of lobula cortex cells across this boundary region disrupts the pattern of lamina marginal glia which normally provides the stop signal for R1-6 axons.[95] *egghead* encodes a beta4-mannosyltransferase[96] which is involved in Glycosphingolipid biosynthesis. Glycosphingolipids have been implicated in EGFR signaling in *Drosophila*.[97]

Selecting the Correct Medulla Target Layer

In the medulla the visual information channels fed by R1-6 are relayed via lamina neuron processes to higher order interneurons. In addition, photoreceptors R7/8 terminate and form synapses exclusively in the medulla (Fig. 7A), where therefore the color vision circuit is predicted to reside[9,19] (Fig. 3). Layering of the medulla reflects the requirement for the establishment of visuotopically organized synapses between these different sets of columnar neurons. In the adult optic lobe the five lamina monopolar neurons and R7 and R8 terminate in different layers of the distal medulla.[18] This enables them to relay on characteristic sets of higher order columnar neurons which project to the lobula complex, most importantly onto transmedulla cells (Tm) projecting to the lobula and transmedulla Y cells (TmY), the axons of which branch in the inner optic chiasm and terminate in lobula and lobula plate (Fig. 2). By inspection of R8 and R7 targeting it was shown that the adult situation is established in an at least two-staged layer-selection process[98] (Fig. 5). During early pupal development the newest leading R8 axon terminates superficially in the distal medulla neuropile and is overtaken by the following R7 axon that temporarily occupies the immediate adjacent deeper layer. These temporary layers of R8 and R7 are more and more pushed apart by the growth cones of the five lamina monopolar cells, which follow and elaborate their arborizations in the space between the R-cell terminals during the first 40% of pupal development. The lamina gradient of maturation from posterior (oldest) to anterior (youngest) is thus reflected as a spatial gradient of the thickness of the medulla in the horizontal plane during early pupal development. At about 50% of pupal development all R7 and R8 growth cones simultaneously become mobile again and target to their final layers M6 and M3.[6,98] The nature of the global trigger of this event is still unknown.

In *sevenless* mutants lacking R7, the axons of R8 and lamina monopolar neurons behave normally during targeting stage I (Fig. 5). The same is true for R8 and R7 terminals in the absence of lamina monopolar neurons. Therefore R8, R7 and L1-L5 axons target independently to their temporary terminal layers at the first layer-selection stage.[98] This layer selection therefore does not seem to depend on interactions between the afferents, but rather on interactions with cells in the target area.

Some factors have been identified that are required for target layer selection. One interesting example is the homophilic cell adhesion protein Capricious (CAPS) with leucine rich repeats, which is present only in R8 and in medulla cells, but not in other retinula cells and not in the lamina.[99] In the medulla neuropil of the third larval instar CAPS is uniformly expressed, but is restricted to specific layers during pupal development sparing the final R7 recipient layer. In flies mutant for *caps*, R-cell terminals in the medulla do not form a regular array and many R8-cell terminals seem to invade neighbouring columns. If CAPS is misexpressed in R7 cells, the first stage of R7 target layer selection is only mildly affected, but the growth cones remain in the final R8 recipient layer. This is evidence that CAPS plays an instructive role in the targeting of R8 terminals.[99]

Other factors required for target layer selection of retinula cells are more widely expressed in the target region and may play a permissive role, e.g., N-cadherin.[6,72] Homophilic cell adhesion mediated by the extracellular domain rather than signaling is important, because the cytoplasmic domain is dispensable not only for N-cadherin mediated cell adhesion in S2 cells but also for targeting of R7 growth cones. However, the cytoplasmic domain is required for normal R7 growth cone morphology.[100] In the lamina, N-cadherin seems to function in a very similar way in the targeting of R1-6 axons as it is expressed and required in the R-cells as well as in the lamina monopolar neurons.[75]

As N-cadherin is not exclusively expressed in specific subsets of neurons in the respective target areas, it is worth mentioning that N-cadherin exists in 12 splice isoforms. In fact, it could be shown that the isoform specific *N-cad* (*18Astop*) allele selectively affects the second stage of R7 target selection.[101] This allele eliminates the six isoforms containing alternative exon 18A. N-cadherin isoforms containing exon 18B are sufficient for the first stage of R7 targeting to its temporary layer, while the 18A isoforms are preferentially expressed in R7 during the second half of pupal development and are necessary for R7 to terminate in the appropriate synaptic layer M6 of the medulla.[101] However, it is very unlikely that the N-cadherin isoforms constitute something like a combinatorial code for the selective recognition of synaptic partners, as expression of any isoform is able to rescue the function of the other and the various isoforms mediate promiscuous heterophilic interactions with each other.[98,101] The function of the structural variations in the isoforms is thus still unknown. It is conceivable that they affect interactions with other proteins rather than homophilic adhesiveness. Therefore N-cadherin can be considered as a homophilic cell adhesion protein providing permissive stabilizing interactions in target selection.

Mutant alleles of the receptor tyrosine phosphatase LAR and its downstream interactor, the scaffolding protein Liprin-α, produce N-cadherin mutant-like targeting defects of R-axons.[74,102-104] Both proteins are expressed like N-cadherin in all R-cells and in neurons of the target areas and their involvement in the regulation of N-cadherin has been shown.[105] However, the requirement of Liprin-α and LAR for R-cell targeting is exclusively on the presynaptic site.[103,104] This implies that N-cadherin regulation is different on the dendritic and on the axonal site. Two heparan sulfate proteoglycans have been identified as ligands for LAR: Dally-like and Syndecan. Both have been implicated in LAR-dependent axon guidance: Syndecan as a promotor and Dally-like as an inhibitor of LAR signaling.[106-108]

The G-protein coupled, 7-pass transmembrane receptor Flamingo is an atypical cadherin, which has recently been shown to regulate synaptogenesis at the neuromuscular junction. In addition, Flamingo is required to prevent axonal and synaptic degeneration in *Drosophila*.[109] Its involvement in optic lobe development is also well established.[73,110,111] Mutations in the *flamingo (fmi)* gene have been discovered in screens for abnormal R-cell connectivity[111] and for defects in visual behaviour.[73] While Flamingo is required for the sorting of R1-6 terminals to their correct lamina cartridges, it has at least two important functions during R8 axon targeting as well: it facilitates competitive interactions between adjacent R8 axons to ensure their correct spacing[73,111] and it promotes the formation of stable connections between R8 axons and their target cells in the medulla.[110,111] The tiling function of Flamingo is not restricted to axonal projections. In other systems, it has been shown to function in the shaping of dendritic fields as well[112] and it was recently shown that ingrowing R8 axons induce layer-specific expression of Flamingo in the medulla via Jelly belly (Jeb) signaling.[110] Its receptor, the anaplastic lymphoma kinase (Alk), is expressed and required in target neurons in the optic lobe. Jeb is generated by photoreceptor axons and controls target selection of R1-R6 axons in the lamina and R8 axons in the medulla. Loss of Jeb/Alk function affects medulla layer-specific expression not only of Flamingo, but also of two cell-adhesion molecules of the immunoglobulin superfamily, Roughest/IrreC and Kirre/Dumbfounded.[110] These closely related single pass transmembrane proteins are known from their function in muscle fusion,[113,114] eye development[27,115] and optic chiasm formation.[116-118] Loss of Roughest/IrreC leads to misrouting via the inner optic chiasm of posterior R8/R7 and lamina monopolar axons to their visuotopic target area.[116] The axonal bundles in the first optic chiasm which connect single lamina cartridges with isotopic medulla columns tend to fasciculate in loss of function mutants,[118] which copies the loss of *flamingo* phenotype in the first chiasm,[73] indicating that the Roughest/IrreC protein helps to keep columnar fibre bundles apart from each other.

Columnar Tiling

While the stratification of columnar neurons reflects their cell type specific connectivity, it is the lateral extent of the arborizations that determines the visuotopic precision of the adult neurons and affects the size and position of their visual fields. It was shown in a classical paper that competition between R7 terminals occurs to a limited degree in the target region.[119] In the third instar, R7 axons transiently display overlapping halos of filopodia, but in genetic mosaics vacant sites are only invaded by neighbouring R7 terminal extensions, if extra R7 axons due to the *more inner photoreceptors* mutation are available in the juxtaposed medulla columns.[119]

The appropriation of territory by neuronal arborizations has at least two aspects. First, the processes of the same neuron have to recognize and arrange themselves. Dendritic as well as axonal arborizations should more or less evenly cover their appropriate target space. Second, neurons of the same type should respect each others territory. The second process is known as "tiling", but the first process is related. It has to be assumed that in both processes recognition of "self" or of "same kind" has to be followed by repulsion. Interestingly homophilic receptors of the conserved family of the Down syndrome cell adhesion molecules (DSCAMs), members of the immunoglobulin superfamily, have been found to function in both aspects of neuronal tiling.[120-122] There are four Dscam genes in the *Drosophila* genome, called Dscam and Dscam2-4. Dscam is special in that it displays an extraordinary molecular diversity. Due to four casettes of alternative spliced exons it can generate 38016 different proteins.[123] Most interestingly, isoform-specific homophilic adhesion seems to induce repulsion in dendrites and thus helps to avoid selfcrossing and contributes to an even coverage of the dendritic field in all four classes of dendrite arborization neurons, a group of sensory neurons with a stereotyped dendritic branching pattern.[120,122] For Dscam2 two isoforms

(Dscam2A and Dscam2B) have been described. They are able to mediate isoform-specific homophilic adhesion in S2-cells and do not bind to other Dscam family members. Dscam2 plays a role in tiling among L1 terminals (Fig. 2A) within the distal medulla. Dscam2 homophilic interactions mediate repulsion between L1 axonal terminals in neighbouring columns. Loss of Dscam2 function leads to an overlap of the L1 terminals.[121]

The repulsive effect of proteins that are able to mediate homophilic adhesion in cell culture experiments demonstrates the importance of signaling for the understanding of cellular responses in vivo. Due to the high number of different types of columnar neurons in the medulla of *Drosophila*[18] it is likely that still other receptors will be described that function in tiling of columnar cell types.

Connecting Optic Lobes with and across the Central Brain

Neuronal connections between the optic lobe and central brain have recently been systematically mapped in considerable detail.[26] Comparably little is known about the development of these projections. Through the study of the transcription factor Atonal, which is originally known to be required for the specification of the R8 ommatidial founder photoreceptor, a dorsal cluster of optic lobe neurons was discovered that connects both optic lobes across the central brain during larval development.[124] The dorsal cluster neurons project contralaterally towards the lobula complex where they fan out over the lobula complex and inner chiasm and additionally form a precise number of projections towards the medulla. This reproducibly accurate projection pattern has been employed to identify an integrative signaling network encompassing the Jun N-terminal kinase, the GTPase Rac, the secreted morphogen Wnt, its receptor Frizzled, the FGF Branchless and the FGF receptor. Importantly, this network regulates the extension and retraction of axonal branches, but not axon guidance, indicating that these processes are regulated independently.[125] Finally, the dorsal cluster neuron projections have also been shown to form independent of neuronal activity, further supporting the notion that wiring of the optic lobes, from cellular differentiation down to the specification of synapses, follow a genetic program.[71,125]

Concluding Remarks

While many steps in optic lobe development are still not yet understood, it is clear that a combination of timing of neuronal and glial cell fate specification, axonal outgrowth, of inductive events and of specific recognition processes between "self" and "not self" direct the wiring of the neural machinery of the optic lobe. It is therefore a genetically encoded developmental program that ensures all aspects of vision required for the survival of the newly emerging fly. Adult optic lobe development is optimized for speed and precision. However, the adult optic lobe also displays a certain degree of plasticity. Deprivation of visual input after the optic lobe is formed can lead to a reduction in synapse numbers in the lamina during a critical time window in early adulthood.[80] However, such plasticity is apparently not required to wire a functional optic lobe. It is therefore an important realization that a brain structure like the *Drosophila* optic lobe is as much the product of a genetically encoded developmental program as the eye or a wing. Given the rich genetic tool box available and the wealth of knowledge about *Drosophila* development, the optic lobe is a wonderful model system to decipher this developmental program and attain knowledge about the extend to which a brain structure can be "genetically encoded".

Acknowlegements

We thank Gerhard Technau for his encouragement throughout the process of writing. KFF thanks the SFB505. PRH is a Eugene McDermott Scholar in Biomedical Research at UT Southwestern Medical Center in Dallas. We thank Claude Desplan and Bassem Hassan for comments on parts of the manuscript. Till Andlauer provided MARCM data. We apologize to all colleagues whose work was not discussed due to space constraints or our shortcomings.

References

1. Green P, Hartenstein AY, Hartenstein V. The embryonic development of the Drosophila visual system. Cell Tissue Res 1993; 273(3):583-598.
2. Meinertzhagen IA, Hanson TE. The development of the optic lobe. In: Bate M, Martinez-Arias A, eds. The Development of Drosophila melanogaster. Cold Spring Harbor: Cold Spring Harbor Press, 1993:1363-1491.
3. Nassif C, Noveen A, Hartenstein V. Early development of the Drosophila brain: III. The pattern of neuropile founder tracts during the larval period. J Comp Neurol 2003; 455(4):417-434.
4. Clandinin TR, Zipursky SL. Making connections in the fly visual system. Neuron 2002; 35(5):827-841.
5. Mast JD, Prakash S, Chen PL et al. The mechanisms and molecules that connect photoreceptor axons to their targets in Drosophila. Semin Cell Dev Biol 2006; 17(1):42-49.
6. Ting CY, Lee CH. Visual circuit development in Drosophila. Curr Opin Neurobiol 2007; 17(1):65-72.
7. Cajal SR, Sanchez D. Contribucion al concocimiento delos centros nerviosos de los insectos. Trab Lab Invest Biol 1915; 13:1-167.
8. Strausfeld NJ. Golgi studies on insects. Part II: The optic lobes of Diptera. Philos Trans R Soc Lond B 1970; 258:135-223.
9. Morante J, Desplan C. Building a projection map for photoreceptor neurons in the Drosophila optic lobes. Semin Cell Dev Biol 2004; 15(1):137-143.
10. Wernet MF, Mazzoni EO, Celik A et al. Stochastic spineless expression creates the retinal mosaic for colour vision. Nature 2006; 440(7081):174-180.
11. Tomlinson A. Patterning the peripheral retina of the fly: decoding a gradient. Dev Cell 2003; 5(5):799-809.
12. Wernet MF, Labhart T, Baumann F et al. Homothorax switches function of Drosophila photoreceptors from color to polarized light sensors. Cell 2003; 115(3):267-279.
13. Homberg U, Hofer S, Pfeiffer K et al. Organization and neural connections of the anterior optic tubercle in the brain of the locust, Schistocerca gregaria. J Comp Neurol 2003; 462(4):415-430.
14. Braitenberg V. Pattern of projections in the visual system of the fly. I. Retina lamina projections. Exp Brain Res 1967; 3:271-298.
15. Kirschfeld K. The projection of the optical environment on the screen of the rhabdomere in the compound eye of Musca. Exp Brain Res 1967; 3:248-270.
16. Trujillo-Cenoz O, Melamed J. Electron microscope observations on the peripheral and intermediate retinas of dipterans. In: Bernhad CG, ed. The Functional Organization of the Compound Eye. New York: Pergamon Press, 1966:339-361.
17. Clandinin TR, Zipursky SL. Afferent growth cone interactions control synaptic specificity in the Drosophila visual system. Neuron 2000; 28(2):427-436.
18. Fischbach K, Dittrich AP. The optic lobe of Drosophila melanogaster. I. A Golgi analysis of wild type structure. Cell Tissue Res 1989; 256:441-475.
19. Bausenwein B, Dittrich AP, Fischbach KF. The optic lobe of Drosophila melanogaster. II. Sorting of retinotopic pathways in the medulla. Cell Tissue Res 1992; 267(1):17-28.
20. Buchner E, Buchner S. Mapping stimulus-induced nervous activity in small brains by [3H]2-deoxy-D-glucose. Cell Tissue Res 1980; 211(1):51-64.
21. Bausenwein B, Fischbach KF. Activity labeling patterns in the medulla of Drosophila melanogaster caused by motion stimuli. Cell Tissue Res 1992; 270(1):25-35.
22. Fischbach K, Ramos RG, Bausenwein B. Der optische Lobus von Drosophila melanogaster: Experimentelle Ansaetze zum Studium von Struktur, Funktion und Entwicklung. Verh Dtsch Zool Ges 1992; 85.2:133-148.
23. Stocker RF. The organization of the chemosensory system in Drosophila melanogaster: a review. Cell Tissue Res 1994; 275(1):3-26.
24. Stocker RF, Lienhard MC, Borst A et al. Neuronal architecture of the antennal lobe in Drosophila melanogaster. Cell Tissue Res 1990; 262(1):9-34.
25. Campos AR, Fischbach KF, Steller H. Survival of photoreceptor neurons in the compound eye of Drosophila depends on connections with the optic ganglia. Development 1992; 114(2):355-366.
26. Otsuna H, Ito K. Systematic analysis of the visual projection neurons of Drosophila melanogaster. I. Lobula-specific pathways. J Comp Neurol 2006; 497(6):928-958.
27. Wolff T, Ready DF. Pattern formation in the Drosophila retina. In: Bate M, Martinez-Arias A, eds. The Development of Drosophila melanogaster. Cold Spring Harbor: Cold Spring Harbor Press, 1993:1363-1491.
28. Murakami S, Umetsu D, Maeyama Y et al. Focal adhesion kinase controls morphogenesis of the Drosophila optic stalk. Development 2007; 134(8):1539-1548.

29. Hofbauer A, Buchner E. Does Drosophila have seven eyes? Naturwissenschaften 1989; 76:335-336.
30. Helfrich-Forster C, Edwards T, Yasuyama K et al. The extraretinal eyelet of Drosophila: development, ultrastructure and putative circadian function. J Neurosci 2002; 22(21):9255-9266.
31. Song J, Wu L, Chen Z et al. Axons guided by insulin receptor in Drosophila visual system. Science 2003; 300(5618):502-505.
32. Garrity PA, Rao Y, Salecker I et al. Drosophila photoreceptor axon guidance and targeting requires the dreadlocks SH2/SH3 adapter protein. Cell 1996; 85(5):639-650.
33. Hing H, Xiao J, Harden N et al. Pak functions downstream of Dock to regulate photoreceptor axon guidance in Drosophila. Cell 25 1999; 97(7):853-863.
34. Houalla T, Hien Vuong D, Ruan W et al. The Ste20-like kinase misshapen functions together with Bicaudal-D and dynein in driving nuclear migration in the developing drosophila eye. Mech Dev 2005; 122(1):97-108.
35. Newsome TP, Schmidt S, Dietzl G et al. Trio combines with dock to regulate Pak activity during photoreceptor axon pathfinding in Drosophila. Cell 2000; 101(3):283-294.
36. Ruan W, Long H, Vuong DH et al. Bifocal is a downstream target of the Ste20-like serine/threonine kinase misshapen in regulating photoreceptor growth cone targeting in Drosophila. Neuron 2002; 36(5):831-842.
37. Ruan W, Pang P, Rao Y. The SH2/SH3 adaptor protein dock interacts with the Ste20-like kinase misshapen in controlling growth cone motility. Neuron 1999; 24(3):595-605.
38. Chevais S. Sur la structure des yeux implantes de Drosophila melanogaster. Archs Anat Microsc 1937; 33:107-112.
39. Halder G, Callaerts P, Gehring WJ. New perspectives on eye evolution. Curr Opin Genet Dev 1995; 5(5):602-609.
40. Steller H, Fischbach KF, Rubin GM. Disconnected: a locus required for neuronal pathway formation in the visual system of Drosophila. Cell 1987; 50(7):1139-1153.
41. Power ME. The effort of reduction in numbers of ommatidia upon the brain of Drosophila melanogaster. J Exp Zool 1943; 94:33-71.
42. Hinke W. Das relative postembryonale Wachstum der Hirnteile von Culex pipiens, Drosophila melanogaster and Drosophila mutanten. Z. Morph Okol Tiere 1961; 50:81-118.
43. Campos-Ortega JA, Hofbauer A. Proliferation pattern and early differentiation of the optic lobes in Drosophila melanogaster. Roux's Arch Dev Biol 1990; 198:264-274.
44. Selleck SB, Gonzalez C, Glover DM et al. Regulation of the G1-S transition in postembryonic neuronal precursors by axon ingrowth. Nature 1992; 355(6357):253-255.
45. Selleck SB, Steller H. The influence of retinal innervation on neurogenesis in the first optic ganglion of Drosophila. Neuron 1991; 6(1):83-99.
46. Winberg ML, Perez SE, Steller H. Generation and early differentiation of glial cells in the first optic ganglion of Drosophila melanogaster. Development 1992; 115(4):903-911.
47. Huang Z, Shilo BZ, Kunes S. A retinal axon fascicle uses spitz, an EGF receptor ligand, to construct a synaptic cartridge in the brain of Drosophila. Cell 1998; 95(5):693-703.
48. Huang Z, Kunes S. Hedgehog, transmitted along retinal axons, triggers neurogenesis in the developing visual centers of the Drosophila brain. Cell 1996; 86(3):411-422.
49. Huang Z, Kunes S. Signals transmitted along retinal axons in Drosophila: Hedgehog signal reception and the cell circuitry of lamina cartridge assembly. Development 1998; 125(19):3753-3764.
50. Chu T, Chiu M, Zhang E et al. A C-terminal motif targets Hedgehog to axons, coordinating assembly of the Drosophila eye and brain. Dev Cell 2006; 10(5):635-646.
51. Chotard C, Leung W, Salecker I. glial cells missing and gcm2 cell autonomously regulate both glial and neuronal development in the visual system of Drosophila. Neuron 2005; 48(2):237-251.
52. Nakato H, Futch TA, Selleck SB. The division abnormally delayed (dally) gene: a putative integral membrane proteoglycan required for cell division patterning during postembryonic development of the nervous system in Drosophila. Development 1995; 121(11):3687-3702.
53. Takeo S, Akiyama T, Firkus C et al. Expression of a secreted form of Dally, a Drosophila glypican, induces overgrowth phenotype by affecting action range of Hedgehog. Dev Biol 2005; 284(1):204-218.
54. Dickson B, Hafen E. Genetic dissection of eye development in drosophila. In: Bate M, Martinez-Arias A, eds. The Development of Drosophila melanogaster. Cold Spring Harbor: Cold Spring Harbor Press, 1993:1363-1491.
55. Dearborn R, He Q, Kunes S et al. Eph receptor tyrosine kinase-mediated formation of a topographic map in the Drosophila visual system. J Neurosci 2002; 22(4):1338-1349.
56. Kunes S, Steller H. Topography in the Drosophila visual system. Curr Opin Neurobiol 1993; 3(1):53-59.
57. Sato M, Umetsu D, Murakami S et al. DWnt4 regulates the dorsoventral specificity of retinal projections in the Drosophila melanogaster visual system. Nat Neurosci 2006; 9(1):67-75.

58. Martin KA, Poeck B, Roth H et al. Mutations disrupting neuronal connectivity in the Drosophila visual system. Neuron 1995; 14(2):229-240.
59. Poeck B, Fischer S, Gunning D et al. Glial cells mediate target layer selection of retinal axons in the developing visual system of Drosophila. Neuron 2001; 29(1):99-113.
60. Yoshida S, Soustelle L, Giangrande A et al. DPP signaling controls development of the lamina glia required for retinal axon targeting in the visual system of Drosophila. Development 2005; 132(20):4587-4598.
61. Frohlich A, Meinertzhagen IA. Synaptogenesis in the first optic neuropile of the fly's visual system. J Neurocytol 1982; 11(1):159-180.
62. Frohlich A, Meinertzhagen IA. Quantitative features of synapse formation in the fly's visual system. I. The presynaptic photoreceptor terminal. J Neurosci 1983; 3(11):2336-2349.
63. Garrity PA, Lee CH, Salecker I et al. Retinal axon target selection in Drosophila is regulated by a receptor protein tyrosine phosphatase. Neuron 1999; 22(4):707-717.
64. Newsome TP, Asling B, Dickson BJ. Analysis of Drosophila photoreceptor axon guidance in eye-specific mosaics. Development 2000; 127:851-860.
65. Gibbs SM, Truman JW. Nitric oxide and cyclic GMP regulate retinal patterning in the optic lobe of Drosophila. Neuron 1998; 20(1):83-93.
66. Rao Y, Pang P, Ruan W et al. brakeless is required for photoreceptor growth-cone targeting in Drosophila. Proc Natl Acad Sci USA 2000; 97(11):5966-5971.
67. Senti K, Keleman K, Eisenhaber F et al. brakeless is required for lamina targeting of R1-R6 axons in the Drosophila visual system. Development 2000; 127(11):2291-2301.
68. Kaminker JS, Canon J, Salecker I et al. Control of photoreceptor axon target choice by transcriptional repression of Runt. Nat Neurosci 2002; 5(8):746-750.
69. Tayler TD, Garrity PA. Axon targeting in the Drosophila visual system. Curr Opin Neurobiol 2003; 13(1):90-95.
70. Zelhof AC, Hardy RW, Becker A et al. Transforming the architecture of compound eyes. Nature 2006; 443(7112):696-699.
71. Hiesinger PR, Zhai RG, Zhou Y et al. Activity-independent prespecification of synaptic partners in the visual map of Drosophila. Curr Biol 2006; 16(18):1835-1843.
72. Lee CH, Herman T, Clandinin TR et al. N-cadherin regulates target specificity in the Drosophila visual system. Neuron 2001; 30(2):437-450.
73. Lee RC, Clandinin TR, Lee CH et al. The protocadherin Flamingo is required for axon target selection in the Drosophila visual system. Nat Neurosci 2003; 6(6):557-563.
74. Maurel-Zaffran C, Suzuki T, Gahmon G et al. Cell-autonomous and -nonautonomous functions of LAR in R7 photoreceptor axon targeting. Neuron 2001; 32(2):225-235.
75. Prakash S, Caldwell JC, Eberl DF et al. Drosophila N-cadherin mediates an attractive interaction between photoreceptor axons and their targets. Nat Neurosci 2005; 8(4):443-450.
76. Hiesinger PR, Reiter C, Schau H et al. Neuropil pattern formation and regulation of cell adhesion molecules in Drosophila optic lobe development depend on synaptobrevin. J Neurosci 1999; 19(17):7548-7556.
77. Mehta SQ, Hiesinger PR, Beronja S et al. Mutations in Drosophila sec15 reveal a function in neuronal targeting for a subset of exocyst components. Neuron 2005; 46(2):219-232.
78. Katz LC, Shatz CJ. Synaptic activity and the construction of cortical circuits. Science 1996; 274(5290):1133-1138.
79. Shatz CJ. Emergence of order in visual system development. Proc Natl Acad Sci USA 1996; 93(2):602-608.
80. Barth M, Hirsch HV, Meinertzhagen IA et al. Experience-dependent developmental plasticity in the optic lobe of Drosophila melanogaster. J Neurosci 1997; 17(4):1493-1504.
81. Bloomquist BT, Shortridge RD, Schneuwly S et al. Isolation of a putative phospholipase C gene of Drosophila, norpA and its role in phototransduction. Cell 1988; 54(5):723-733.
82. Burg MG, Sarthy PV, Koliantz G et al. Genetic and molecular identification of a Drosophila histidine decarboxylase gene required in photoreceptor transmitter synthesis. EMBO J 1993; 12(3):911-919.
83. Hardie RC. Is histamine a neurotransmitter in insect photoreceptors? J Comp Physiol [A] 1987; 161(2):201-213.
84. Koh TW, Bellen HJ. Synaptotagmin I, a Ca2+ sensor for neurotransmitter release. Trends Neurosci 2003; 26(8):413-422.
85. Meinertzhagen IA, Hu X. Evidence for site selection during synaptogenesis: the surface distribution of synaptic sites in photoreceptor terminals of the files Musca and Drosophila. Cell Mol Neurobiol 1996; 16(6):677-698.
86. Meinertzhagen IA, Sorra KE. Synaptic organization in the fly's optic lamina: few cells, many synapses and divergent microcircuits. Prog Brain Res 2001; 131:53-69.

87. Frohlich A, Meinertzhagen IA. Regulation of synaptic frequency: comparison of the effects of hypoinnervation with those of hyperinnervation in the fly's compound eye. J Neurobiol 1987; 18(4):343-357.
88. Strausfeld NJ. Atlas of an Insect Brain. Heidelberg: Springer Verlag; 1976.
89. Strausfeld NJ, Okamura JY. Visual system of calliphorid flies: organization of optic glomeruli and their lobula complex efferents. J Comp Neurol 2007; 500(1):166-188.
90. Fischbach KF, Heisenberg M. Structural brain mutant of Drosophila melanogaster with reduced cell number in the medulla cortex and with normal optomotor yaw response. Proc Natl Acad Sci USA 1981; 78(2):1105-1109.
91. Fischbach KF. Neural cell types surviving congenital sensory deprivation in the optic lobes of Drosophila melanogaster. Dev Biol 1983; 95(1):1-18.
92. Fischbach KF, Technau G. Cell degeneration in the developing optic lobes of the sine oculis and small-optic-lobes mutants of Drosophila melanogaster. Dev Biol 1984; 104(1):219-239.
93. Younossi-Hartenstein A, Salvaterra PM, Hartenstein V. Early development of the Drosophila brain: IV. Larval neuropile compartments defined by glial septa. J Comp Neurol 2003; 455(4):435-450.
94. Tayler TD, Robichaux MB, Garrity PA. Compartmentalization of visual centers in the Drosophila brain requires Slit and Robo proteins. Development 2004; 131(23):5935-5945.
95. Fan Y, Soller M, Flister S et al. The egghead gene is required for compartmentalization in Drosophila optic lobe development. Dev Biol 2005; 287(1):61-73.
96. Wandall HH, Pizette S, Pedersen JW et al. Egghead and brainiac are essential for glycosphingolipid biosynthesis in vivo. J Biol Chem 2005; 280(6):4858-4863.
97. Chen YW, Pedersen JW, Wandall HH et al. Glycosphingolipids with extended sugar chain have specialized functions in development and behavior of Drosophila. Dev Biol 2007; 306(2):736-749.
98. Ting CY, Yonekura S, Chung P et al. Drosophila N-cadherin functions in the first stage of the two-stage layer-selection process of R7 photoreceptor afferents. Development 2005; 132(5):953-963.
99. Shinza-Kameda M, Takasu E, Sakurai K et al. Regulation of layer-specific targeting by reciprocal expression of a cell adhesion molecule, capricious. Neuron 2006; 49(2):205-213.
100. Yonekura S, Xu L, Ting CY et al. Adhesive but not signaling activity of Drosophila N-cadherin is essential for target selection of photoreceptor afferents. Dev Biol 2007; 304(2):759-770.
101. Nern A, Nguyen LV, Herman T et al. An isoform-specific allele of Drosophila N-cadherin disrupts a late step of R7 targeting. Proc Natl Acad Sci USA 2005; 102(36):12944-12949.
102. Clandinin TR, Lee CH, Herman T et al. Drosophila LAR regulates R1-R6 and R7 target specificity in the visual system. Neuron 2001; 32(2):237-248.
103. Choe KM, Prakash S, Bright A et al. Liprin-alpha is required for photoreceptor target selection in Drosophila. Proc Natl Acad Sci USA 2006; 103(31):11601-11606.
104. Hofmeyer K, Maurel-Zaffran C, Sink H et al. Liprin-alpha has LAR-independent functions in R7 photoreceptor axon targeting. Proc Natl Acad Sci USA 2006; 103(31):11595-11600.
105. Kypta RM, Su H, Reichardt LF. Association between a transmembrane protein tyrosine phosphatase and the cadherin-catenin complex. J Cell Biol 1996; 134(6):1519-1529.
106. Fox AN, Zinn K. The heparan sulfate proteoglycan syndecan is an in vivo ligand for the Drosophila LAR receptor tyrosine phosphatase. Curr Biol 2005; 15(19):1701-1711.
107. Rawson JM, Dimitroff B, Johnson KG et al. The heparan sulfate proteoglycans Dally-like and Syndecan have distinct functions in axon guidance and visual-system assembly in Drosophila. Curr Biol 2005; 15(9):833-838.
108. Johnson KG, Tenney AP, Ghose A et al. The HSPGs Syndecan and Dallylike bind the receptor phosphatase LAR and exert distinct effects on synaptic development. Neuron 2006; 49(4):517-531.
109. Bao H, Berlanga ML, Xue M et al. The atypical cadherin flamingo regulates synaptogenesis and helps prevent axonal and synaptic degeneration in Drosophila. Mol Cell Neurosci 2007; 34(4):662-678.
110. Bazigou E, Apitz H, Johansson J et al. Anterograde Jelly belly and Alk receptor tyrosine kinase signaling mediates retinal axon targeting in Drosophila. Cell 2007; 128(5):961-975.
111. Senti KA, Usui T, Boucke K et al. Flamingo regulates R8 axon-axon and axon-target interactions in the Drosophila visual system. Curr Biol 2003; 13(10):828-832.
112. Kimura H, Usui T, Tsubouchi A et al. Potential dual molecular interaction of the Drosophila 7-pass transmembrane cadherin Flamingo in dendritic morphogenesis. J Cell Sci 2006; 119(Pt 6):1118-1129.
113. Ruiz-Gomez M, Coutts N, Price A et al. Drosophila dumbfounded: a myoblast attractant essential for fusion. Cell 2000; 102(2):189-198.
114. Strunkelnberg M, Bonengel B, Moda LM et al. rst and its paralogue kirre act redundantly during embryonic muscle development in Drosophila. Development 2001; 128(21):4229-4239.
115. Reiter C, Schimansky T, Nie Z et al. Reorganization of membrane contacts prior to apoptosis in the Drosophila retina: the role of the IrreC-rst protein. Development 1996; 122(6):1931-1940.
116. Boschert U, Ramos RG, Tix S et al. Genetic and developmental analysis of irreC, a genetic function required for optic chiasm formation in Drosophila. J Neurogenet 1990; 6(3):153-171.

117. Ramos RG, Igloi GL, Lichte B et al. The irregular chiasm C-roughest locus of Drosophila, which affects axonal projections and programmed cell death, encodes a novel immunoglobulin-like protein. Genes Dev 1993; 7(12B):2533-2547.
118. Schneider T, Reiter C, Eule E et al. Restricted expression of the irreC-rst protein is required for normal axonal projections of columnar visual neurons. Neuron 1995; 15(2):259-271.
119. Ashley JA, Katz FN. Competition and position-dependent targeting in the development of the Drosophila R7 visual projections. Development 1994; 120(6):1537-1547.
120. Hughes ME, Bortnick R, Tsubouchi A et al. Homophilic Dscam interactions control complex dendrite morphogenesis. Neuron 2007; 54(3):417-427.
121. Millard SS, Flanagan JJ, Pappu KS et al. Dscam2 mediates axonal tiling in the Drosophila visual system. Nature 2007; 447(7145):720-724.
122. Soba P, Zhu S, Emoto K et al. Drosophila sensory neurons require Dscam for dendritic self-avoidance and proper dendritic field organization. Neuron 2007; 54(3):403-416.
123. Schmucker D, Clemens JC, Shu H et al. Drosophila Dscam is an axon guidance receptor exhibiting extraordinary molecular diversity. Cell 2000; 101(6):671-684.
124. Hassan BA, Bermingham NA, He Y et al. Atonal regulates neurite arborization but does not act as a proneural gene in the Drosophila brain. Neuron 2000; 25(3):549-561.
125. Srahna M, Leyssen M, Choi CM et al. A signaling network for patterning of neuronal connectivity in the Drosophila brain. PLoS Biol 2006; 4(11):e348.
126. Fischbach KF. Neurogenetik am Beispiel des visuellen Systems von Drosophila melanogaster.: Habilitationsschrift. Bayerische Julius-Maximilians-Universität Würzburg; 1983.
127. Jarvilehto M, Finell N. Development of the function of visual receptor cells during the pupal life of the fly Calliphora. J Comp Physiol [A] 1983; 150:529-536.
128. Hardie RC, Peretz A, Pollock JA et al. Ca2+ limits the development of the light response in Drosophila photoreceptors. Proc Biol Sci 1993; 252(1335):223-229.
129. Meinertzhagen IA, Piper ST, Sun XJ et al. Neurite morphogenesis of identified visual interneurons and its relationship to photoreceptor synaptogenesis in the flies, Musca domestica and Drosophila melanogaster. Eur J Neurosci 2000; 12(4):1342-1356.

Clonal Unit Architecture of the Adult Fly Brain

Kei Ito* and Takeshi Awasaki

Abstract

During larval neurogenesis, neuroblasts repeat asymmetric cell divisions to generate clonally related progeny. When the progeny of a single neuroblast is visualized in the larval brain, their cell bodies form a cluster and their neurites form a tight bundle. This structure persists in the adult brain. Neurites deriving from the cells in this cluster form bundles to innervate distinct areas of the brain. Such clonal unit structure was first identified in the mushroom body, which is formed by four nearly identical clonal units each of which consists of diverse types of neurons. Organised structures in other areas of the brain, such as the central complex and the antennal lobe projection neurons, also consist of distinct clonal units. Many clonally related neural circuits are observed also in the rest of the brain, which is often called diffused neuropiles because of the apparent lack of clearly demarcated structures. Thus, it is likely that the clonal units are the building blocks of a significant portion of the adult brain circuits. Arborisations of the clonal units are not mutually exclusive, however. Rather, several clonal units contribute together to form distinct neural circuit units, to which other clones contribute relatively marginally. Construction of the brain by combining such groups of clonally related units would have been a simple and efficient strategy for building the complicated neural circuits during development as well as during evolution.

Introduction

The fly brain consists of a complicated meshwork of neural circuits.[1,2] Each neuron projects to and arborises in its distinct subareas. Visualisation of specific subtypes of neurons, either by antibody staining or by expression of reporter genes, suggests that, although certain variability is observed in the number of the labelled cells, the projection patterns of the labelled neurons are rather stereotyped in the adult brain.[3-5] Molecular mechanisms underlying the formation of such complicated but stereotyped neural architecture have been studied extensively during the past few decades. Neurons are generated by asymmetric division of the stem cells called neuroblasts.[6,7] Each neuroblast gives birth to a series of clonal progeny during neurogenesis. The brain is therefore composed of "families" of clonally related cells. In this chapter, we examine how such lineage-dependent groups of neurons contribute to the formation of the elaborated neural circuits of the adult fly brain.

Structure of the Adult Brain

Before discussing the relationship between clones and neural network, we will briefly overview the general structure of the adult fly brain (for structure and development of the larval brain, see chapter by V Hartenstein et al). The adult brain is a mass of neurons that is about 500 μm wide, 200 μm thick and 250 μm tall. It consists of three parts, the central brain and an optic lobe on either side. The latter is the lower-order sensory centre specialised for visual information processing,[8,9] whereas the former contains lower-order centres of other sensory modalities (olfactory,

*Corresponding Author: Kei Ito—Institute of Molecular and Cellular Biosciences, the University of Tokyo, Yayoi, Bunkyo-ku, Tokyo 113-0032, Japan. Email: itokei@iam.u-tokyo.ac.jp

Brain Development in Drosophila melanogaster, edited by Gerhard M. Technau.
©2008 Landes Bioscience and Springer Science+Business Media.

etc.) as well as integrative and associative centres and higher-order motor control centres. Figures 1A,B show sections of a silver-stained adult fly brain. The area near the brain surface is occupied by the rind, or cortex, where cell bodies of all the neurons are confined (yellow areas). Unlike vertebrates, insect neurons have no synapses around their cell bodies. Thus, there are no synapses in the rind. All the brain neurons are monopolar, sending single neurites (cell body fibres) deeper into the brain and form synaptic connections[2] (Fig. 1C). The area occupied by these fibres and synapses is called the neuropile.

The thickness of the rind is different depending on the area of the brain. It is thickest in the area called the lateral cell body region (LCBR), which is between the central brain and the optic lobe (Fig. 1A,B). The rind is thin in the areas where the underlying neuropiles are protruded. Especially, there are essentially no cell bodies in the anteriormost surface area of the suboesophageal ganglion (SOG), antennal lobe (AL), ventrolateral protocerebrum (vlpr) and the anterior inferiorlateral protocerebrum (aimpr) (Fig. 1D). The ventral area of the posterior brain has no cell bodies, either, because this area is occupied by the cervical connective that houses the descending and ascending neural fibres to and from the thoracic ganglion (Fig. 1E). The diameter of the neural cell bodies tend to be smaller in the optic lobe and in the area above the calyx (ca) of the mushroom body (MB) than in other areas of the central brain (Fig. 1E).

Neurites generally form arborisations in several areas along their trajectories (Fig. 1C). The arborisations that are closest from the cell bodies are called the primary arborisations and those that are farthest are the terminal arborisations. In a simplistic view, the primary arborisation is often regarded as "postsynaptic dendrites" or "input areas," whereas the terminal arborisation is often called "presynaptic axon terminals" or "output areas." Though this is true in some cases, the situation is often more complicated. For example, many projection neurons that convey olfactory information from the AL to the second-order olfactory centres (the MB and the lateral horn, LH) have presynaptic sites not only in their terminals in the MB and LH but also in their dendrites in the AL (R Okada and KI, unpublished observation). Kenyon cells of the MB have postsynaptic sites not only in the calyx, which is supposed to be the input area of the MB, but also in the lobes, which is regarded as its output area.[10] Thus, pre and postsynaptic sites may in various cases co-exist in the same branches of neurites. Presynaptic sites in the primary arborisations may function for emitting local feedback signals and postsynaptic sites in the terminal arborisations might receive local modification signals for their output. On the other hand, there are indeed some neurons in which pre and postsynaptic sites are preferentially distributed in the proximal and distal areas of the neurites, respectively.[8] The direction of information therefore is not self evident from the projection pattern alone. Because the term "dendrite" often infers its role as input sites, care should be taken when using this word for referring to certain primary arborisations.

The brain consists of neurons and glial cells. Figure 1F,G show cross sections of the brain labelled for synaptic areas (with monoclonal antibody nc82[11]) and glial processes (with GFP driven by the glial specific repo-GAL4 driver.) The rind is contributed extensively by the processes of cell body glia (or cortex glia),[12] which ensheath each neural cell body. As explained before, synapses exist only in the neuropile. By comparing Figure 1A and 1G, which show the sections of the same level of the brain, it is clear that the neuropile areas that are occupied by large tracts of neural fibres (bundles of thick lines in Fig. 1A) are devoid of synapses (black areas in Fig. 1G). These tracts are covered by the processes of the neuropile glial cells.

The neuropile glia also separate the borders between major brain areas. For example, the borders around the AL, MB and the central complex, as well as the border between the suboesophageal ganglion (SOG) and the supraoesophageal ganglion, are covered by the glial sheath. Glial processes, however, do not always demarcate borders between functional areas of the neuropile. For example, although the MB is covered extensively by glial processes, there is no glial sheath structure between the LH—the other second-order olfactory centre—and the surrounding neuropiles. Similarly, although the anterior half of the ventrolateral protocerebrum (vlpr) is clearly demarcated by glial processes, the border between its posterior half and neighbouring neuropiles is more ambiguous.

Whereas three particular regions of the central brain, the AL, MB and the central complex, have clear glial sheaths that demarcate their borders and simple and organised circuit structures within them, neural fibres in the rest of the central brain do not form clearly distinguishable unit structures. These areas are often collectively called "diffused neuropiles." Short of a comprehensive knowledge about the circuit structures in the diffused neuropiles, it is not possible to determine the functional areas unambiguously in these brain areas. Therefore we here rely on a simple block-based terminology system to describe the subregions in these neuropiles (Fig. 1H-N).[2,5]

The central brain is divided into two parts: the supraoesophageal and suboesophageal ganglia. They are separated clearly in insect species that appeared earlier during evolution, but in flies they are fused with no clear external border (Fig. 1A,D). The supraoesophageal ganglion is divided into three neuromeres, the proto-, deuto- and tritocerebrum. The protocerebrum occupies most area of the supraoesophageal ganglion. The deutocerebrum is a small, flat area that lies beneath the protocerebrum and spans on both sides of the SOG. The neuropiles that receive sensory projections from the antennae, i.e., the AL and the antennal mechanosensory and motor centre (AMMC), are parts of the deutocerebrum (Fig. 1M,N).[13-15] Evolutionary studies and analyses of early embryogenesis suggest that the animal body anterior to the oesophagus is likely to consist of three segments (Chapter 2). Thus, the third supraoesophageal neuromere, the tritocerebrum, should exist somewhere between the deutocerebrum and the SOG. Such neuromere is not clearly discernible in the adult fly brain, however (Fig. 1A,G).

The SOG can also be divided into three neuromeres: the mandibular, maxillary and labial neuromeres. They derive from the three head segments posterior to the oesophagus and each neuromere receives peripheral nerves from the corresponding head segment. The internal borders between these neuromeres within the brain, however, are difficult to identify. The SOG consists mainly of the terminals of sensory neurons from the mouth and the surface of the head capsule and dendrites of the motor neurons for the head muscles. Judging from its primary role that is closely associated with the peripheral nervous systems, the SOG is functionally more similar to the thoracic ganglion than to the supraoesophageal ganglion. For this reason, the term "brain" sometimes refers specifically to the supraoesophageal ganglion.

As this example shows, the definition of the word "brain" is somewhat ambiguous in the insect nervous system (Table 1). Depending on the context, it refers to either all the central nervous system that resides in the head capsule, the supraoesophageal ganglion including the optic lobes, the combination of the SOG and the central part of the supraoesophageal ganglion, or only the central part of the supraoesophageal ganglion. To avoid confusion, in this chapter we use the word "brain" to refer to all the central nervous system in the head and use the words shown in parentheses of Table 1 to refer to each specific part of it.

Techniques for Visualising Clonally Related Progeny

Neuroblasts divide asymmetrically to generate their progeny (Fig. 2A). The proliferation pattern is rather different between the optic lobe and the central brain (inset photograph in Fig. 2A). In the optic lobe, precursor cells arranged in the two optic anlagen first divide symmetrically to increase their number and than asymmetrically, to produce large numbers of progeny[16] (see Chapter by KF Fischbach and PR Hiesinger). In the central brain, the proliferation pattern is essentially the same as in the thoracic ganglion (the ventral nerve cord), where a limited number of neuroblasts

Table 1. Classification of the brain areas

Suboesophageal ganglion	Supraoesophageal ganglion without optic lobe		Optic lobe
	Brain		
SOG	**Brain** (→ *supraoesophageal ganglion*)		
Brain (→ *central brain*)			Optic lobe
SOG	**Brain** (→ *cerebrum*)		Optic lobe

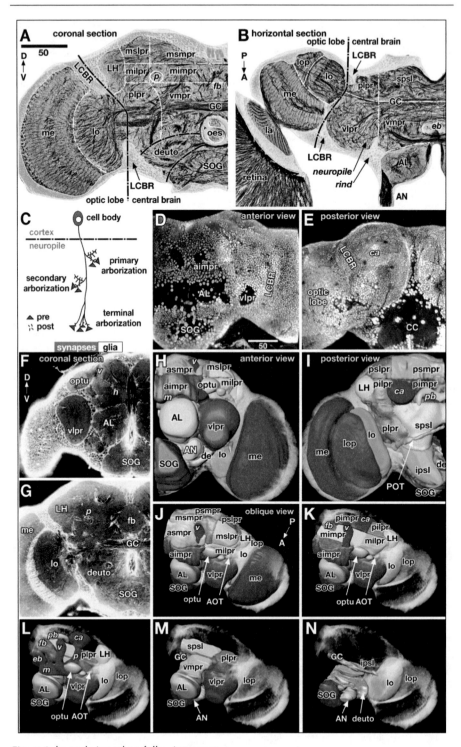

Figure 1, legend viewed on following pages.

Figure 1, viewed on prvious page. Overall structure of the adult fly brain. A,B) Coronal (frontal, A) and horizontal (B) sections of silver-stained brains (A, B, D and N modified from ref. 5 with permission from John Wiley and Sons, Inc. ©2006). Areas with yellow overlay represent the rind, or cortex. Black dashed lines show the border between the central brain and the optic lobe and between neuromeres (A). White lines show the arbitrary border of the neuropile regions. C) Scheme of a neuron in the brain. D,E) Distribution of the neural cell bodies, showing the anterior (D) and posterior (E) views of the brain. Three-dimensional (3D) reconstruction of the confocal optical sections of the brain expressing nuclear-specific reporter UAS-*NLS-lacZ* driven by elav-GAL4 enhancer trap strain c155 (modified from ref. 10). F, G) Confocal optical sections, showing the anterior (F) and middle (G) areas (Data by H. Otsuna). Magenta represents the synaptic areas visualised by the monoclonal antibody nc82, which recognises the active zone protein, Bruchpilot.[11] White represents the glial processes visualised with UAS-*GFP* driven with glia-specific repo-GAL4 driver. H-N) Neuropile regions defined for indicating the positions in the brain (modified from ref. 5). 3D reconstruction of the anterior (H), posterior (I) and anterior-dorsal oblique (J-N) views of the brain showing neuropile regions at different dorsoventral levels. Because analysis of the function and neural architecture of the diffused neuropiles remains scarce and spotty, our current knowledge is not enough for making conclusive regional map that reflects the functional organisation of this area. To provide a way to describe neuropile regions unambiguously under this situation, borders of the neuropile regions are here defined arbitrarily with simple planes that are defined in association with easily recognisable landmarks such as the MB and the great commissure (GC). This nomenclature system is introduced by Strausfeld[2] and expanded by Otsuna and Ito.[5]

List of the neuropile regions: The dorsal area of the protocerebrum is divided into two areas: the superiormedial protocerebrum (smpr) and the superiorlateral protocerebrum (slpr). The sagittal border between smpr and slpr is defined by the lateral surface of the MB pedunculus (p). The horizontal border between the superior protocerebrum and the inferior protocerebrum is defined with the 50% height between the ventral surface of the pedunculus and the tip of the MB vertical lobe. *asmpr* (anterior superiormedial protocerebrum): the asmpr is the anteriormost area of the smpr, between the two vertical lobes (v) of the MB. The area slightly lateral to the MB vertical lobe but dorsomedial to the lateral pedunculus surface is included in the aimpr, because many neurons around the vertical lobe arborise also in its lateral side. The posterior border of the asmpr is defined with the posterior surface of the MB vertical lobe. *msmpr* (middle superiormedial protocerebrum): the middle area of the smpr, directly posterior to the asmpr. Its posterior border is defined with the plane above the GC. The pars intercerebralis—the area near the midline with many large cell bodies of neurosecretory cells—lies in the medialmost region of the msmpr. *psmpr* (posterior superiormedial protocerebrum): the posteriormost area of the smpr, spanning above and anterodorsal to the MB calyx (ca). *mslpr* (middle superiorlateral protocerebrum): the area lateral to the msmpr. Note that there is no area called the aslpr, because there is no neuropile anterolateral to the MB vertical lobe (see Fig. 1J). *pslpr* (posterior superiorlateral protocerebrum): the area lateral to the psmpr, dorsolateral to the MB calyx. The area below the superior protocerebrum and above the ventral surface of the pedunculus is the inferiormedial protocerebrum (impr) and inferiorlateral protocerebrum (ilpr). *aimpr* (anterior inferiormedial protocerebrum): The anteriormost area of the impr, above the antennal lobe and in front of the posterior surface of the MB vertical lobe. The medial lobe of the MB is embedded in this area. *mimpr* (middle inferiormedial protocerebrum): The area of the impr behind the MB lobes, anterior to the plane above the GC and medial to the lateral surface of the pedunculus. The dorsal half of the ellipsoid body (eb) and the fan-shaped body (fb) of the central complex is contained in this area. *pimpr* (posterior inferiormedial protocerebrum): The area between and anteromedial to the calyx. The protocerebral bridge (pb) of the central complex lies in this area. *optu* (optic tubercle): The anteriormost area of the ilpr, lateral to the aimpr. Though this area could be called as ailpr, it is occupied by the structure that is traditionally called as the optic tubercle, which is contributed by the terminals of the visual projection neurons from the optic lobe via the anterior optic tract (AOT). *milpr* (middle inferiorlateral protocerebrum): The area lateral to the mimpr. *pilpr* (posterior inferiorlateral protocerebrum): The area lateral to the pimpr, between the calyx and the lateral horn. *LH* (lateral horn): The area protruded in the lateral area of the central brain, between the milpr and pilpr. This area contains the terminals of the olfactory projection neurons from the AL. *AL* (antennal lobe). Legend continued on following page.

Figure 1, viewed on page 138. The anterior protrusion of the medial cerebrum, receiving projections of the sensory neurons of the antennae via the antennal nerve (AN). It is a part of the deutocerebrum. *vmpr* (ventromedial protocerebrum): The area just posterior to the AL, in front of the GC and ventromedial to the MB pedunculus. Unlike the AL, it is a part of the protocerebrum. It houses the ventral half of the ellipsoid body and the fan-shaped body as well as the lateral accessory lobe (also called the ventral body), an annex of the central complex that is important for motor control. *spsl* (superior posterior slope): Dorsal part of the area in the posterior brain surrounding the oesophagus foramen. It receives projections from the ocellar nerve and is also contributed by the dendrites of descending neurons. *ipsl* (inferior posterior slope): The area of the posterior slope ventral to the oesophagus foramen, which also houses dendrites of descending neurons. *vlpr* (ventrolateral protocerebrum): A large area in the lateral cerebrum in front of the GC. It is also called the anterior optic foci, because it receives many visual projections from the optic lobe. Their terminals in this area form several glomerular structures called the optic glomeruli. *plpr* (posteriorlateral protocerebrum): The area behind the vlpr, which is also called the posterior optic foci. Like vlpr, many visual projection neurons terminate in the plpr. *de* (deutocerebrum): The area posterior ventral to the AL. It houses the antennal mechanosensory and motor centre (AMMC), which receives projections of auditory and mechanosensory neurons from the antennae. The AL is actually also a part of the de. *SOG* (suboesophageal ganglion): The neuromere ventral to the oesophagus. Other labelled structures: *la*: lamina, *me*: medulla, *lo*: lobula, *lop*: lobula plate, *AOT*: anterior optic tract, *POT*: posterior optic tract, *LCBR*: lateral cell body region.

distributed around the surface of the nervous system each generates a large number of neurons.[6,7] Each cell division yields a neuroblast and a ganglion mother cell (GMC). It is generally believed that a GMC divides once more to generate two neural progeny. Most neuroblasts proliferate at two separate periods during neurogenesis.[7] The first proliferation occurs during mid to late embryonic stage, whereas the second proliferation starts from between the late first and late second larval instar and ends during the first day of the pupal stage. Thus, the clonal progeny of most neuroblasts consists of embryonic and postembryonic neurons (Fig. 2A).[17]

In the larval brain, there are about 100 neuroblasts per hemisphere in the cerebrum[7,18,19] and about 80 per hemisphere in the SOG (R Urbach and GM Technau, personal communication). There are therefore in total about 180 neuroblasts in a central brain hemisphere. Counting of cell bodies in the nuclear-labelled brain samples suggests that there are about 18,000 cells per hemisphere in the adult central brain including the SOG (T Shimada and KI, unpublished observation). Considering that some neuroblasts, such as those that generate the MB Kenyon cells, give birth to several hundred progeny,[7] the number of progeny of most other neuroblasts should be less than a hundred.

How, then, does each family of clonally related neurons contribute to the formation of the adult neural circuits? One possibility is that each neuron differentiates and sends its neurites independently from cell lineage (left panel of Fig. 2B). The other possibility is that neurons of a particular clone form distinct subcomponents of the neural circuits (right panel of Fig. 2B).

To determine which is more likely, a technique is required to visualise the projection pattern of all the progeny of one neuroblast in the adult nervous system. This has not been an easy task. Cell lineage can in principle be traced by injecting dyes to a cell early during development.[20-24] Though this worked well for analysing cell lineage in embryos, postembryonic progeny could not be labelled with this technique, because injected dye is diluted below detection level as neuroblasts repeat cell division. To circumvent this problem, transplantation of genetically labelled neuroblasts was developed.[17,25] In this technique, a neuroblast is picked out from an embryo expressing a reporter gene (e.g., *lacZ*) under control of a ubiquitous promoter. The neuroblast is then transplanted to a host embryo that does not carry the reporter gene. Though this system is versatile,[26-28] technical expertise is required for cell transplantation and differences in the cell positions and developmental stages between donor and host embryos might affect subsequent development of the transplanted neuroblast. Thanks to the powerful *Drosophila* genetics, however, several techniques that are easier to label clonally related cells were developed during the last decade. They use genetic mosaic

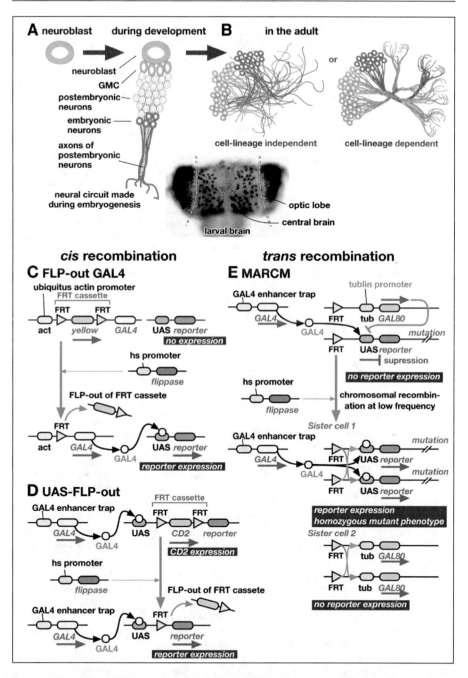

Figure 2. Neuroblast proliferation and techniques for labelling clonally related cells. A) Scheme of the neuroblast and its progeny in the larval brain. *GMC*: ganglion mother cell. Photographic inset: Larval brain shortly before puparium formation. Proliferating cells are labelled with bromodeoxyuridine (BrdU) incorporation by larval feeding and visualised with anti-BrdU antibody. Figure legend continued on next page.

Figure 2, viewed on previous page. B) Two possible strategies for constructing the neural cicuits of the adult brain. C) FLP-out-GAL4 (FRT-GAL4) system. In the first component, a marker gene *yellow* flanked by a pair of FRTs (FRT cassette) is inserted between the ubiquitous actin promoter and the transcription activator *GAL4*. Because there is no promoter directly in front of *GAL4*, only *yellow* is expressed. By applying mild heat shock to the animal during development, the heat-shock (hs) promoter activates the expression of the second component, hs-*flippase*, in some cells. Flippase protein induces recombination between the two FRTs, excising the *yellow* gene between them (FLP-out). In the cells in which this recombination occurred and also in its progeny, the actin promoter starts driving the expression of *GAL4*. The expression of the third component, a reporter gene such as *GFP* under control of the GAL4-target sequence UAS, is activated only in these cells. D) UAS-FLP-out system: The *GAL4* gene is expressed in a cell-type specific manner using certain promoter or GAL4 enhancer-trap strains. The second component features UAS and a reporter gene separated by an FRT cassette containing the *CD2* gene. GAL4 activates the expression of only *CD2*. A mild heat shock activates *flippase*, which excises the FRT cassette. This enables the expression of the reporter gene in the cell and its progeny. E) MARCM system: A ubiquitous tublin promoter drives constitutive expression of yeast-derived *GAL80*, which suppresses expression of the UAS-linked reporter gene even in the presence of *GAL4*. The tublin-*GAL80* and the reporter gene are put in the homologous chromosome in trans and the FRT sequence is put in the locus close to the centromere of each chromosome. Upon mild heat shock, *trans* recombination between two chromosomes occurs in some of the cells during mitosis. One of the daughter cell becomes homozygous for the UAS-reporter. Because GAL80 no longer exists in the genome of this cell and its progeny, the cells are visualised by the reporter.

analysis combined with yeast-derived GAL4-UAS[29-31] and flippase-FRT systems[32-34] and can be categorised into two groups.

cis-*Recombination Systems*

Flippase is the enzyme that induces recombination between two sequences called the flippase recognition targets (FRTs). The first group of techniques label cells by inducing *cis*-recombination between two FRT sequences on the same chromosome. First, a gene or a stop-codon sequence is placed between the two FRTs. This "FRT cassette" is then put between a reporter gene and a promoter of a ubiquitous house-keeping gene, e.g., actin or tublin. Because of the inserted FRT cassette, the ubiquitous promoter cannot drive the expression of the reporter gene. By inducing the expression of *flippase* transiently during development, e.g., by putting the *flippase* gene under the heat-shock promoter and giving temporal heat shock to the transgenic animals, recombination between the two FRTs would occur in some cells. This removes the FRT cassette (flip-out or FLP-out) and connect the ubiquitous promoter and the reporter gene directly. The reporter gene would be expressed specifically in these cells as well as in their progeny. If the recombination occurs in the GMC or in the postmitotic cells, single or a few scattered cells would be labelled. If the recombination occurs in the neuroblast, on the other hand, a group of clonally related cells can be visualised.

Such system was first developed by putting the *lacZ* gene after the FRT cassette.[35] An improved version featured *GAL4* instead of *lacZ*, which can activate the expression of diverse types of reporter genes to visualise different aspects of the labelled cells (FRT-GAL4, or FLP-out GAL4 system, Fig. 2C).[36] Because GAL4 can activate multiple UAS targets, genes that affect the function or development of the cells—so called effector genes—can be expressed simultaneously with the reporter genes, enabling the functional analyses of the expressed genes using this system.

Another approach is to put the FRT cassette between the UAS and the reporter gene (the UAS-FLP-out system, Fig. 2D).[37] This system can be combined with a wide variety of promoter-GAL4 lines and GAL4 enhancer-trap strains currently available, in which GAL4 is expressed specifically in particular cells. Depending on whether the recombination occurred in the neuroblast or in the postmitotic cells, the UAS-FLP-out system visualizes a clonally related subset or the morphology of the single cells out of the *GAL4*-expressing cell population.[15,38]

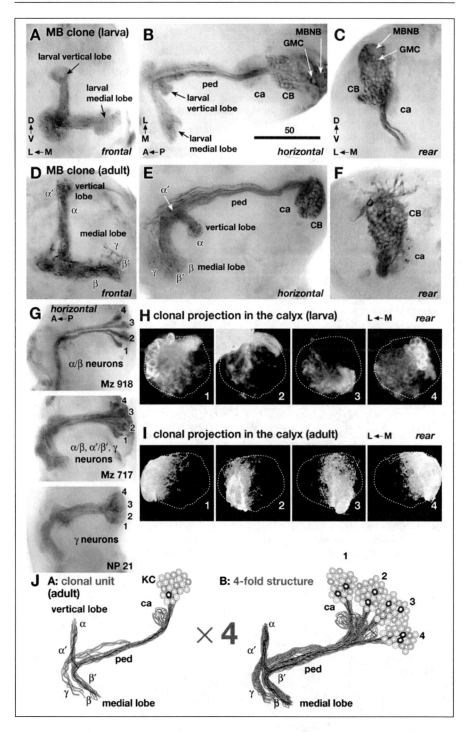

Figure 3, legend viewed on following page.

Figure 3, viewed on previous page. Clonal units in the mushroom body. A-F) A clone labelled in larvae just after hatching and visualised at the end of the larval stage (A-C) and another clone visualised in the adult (D-F), respectively (modified from ref. 36). (FLP-out-GAL4 clones visualised with UAS-*tau* reporter. UAS-*tau* and UAS-*GFP* reporters label essentially similar structures, except that Tau labels dendritic arborisations more weakly and occasionally causes mild disturbance of the neural function.) Optical sections at different levels were taken with Nomarski optics and montaged. Frontal, horizontal and rear views of the same clone was visualized by rotating the specimen. *MBNB*: mushroom body neuroblasts, *CB*: cell bodies, *ca*: calyx, *ped*: pedunculus. G) Four-fold labelling pattern of enhancer-trap strains labelling subsets of the MB Kenyon cells. (Modified from ref. 36, UAS-*tau* reporter). H) Cross section of the calyx in the larval brain, showing areas of arborisations of each of the four clonal units. (Modified from ref. 42, ©2005 National Academy of Sciences, U.S.A., MARCM clone with UAS-*GFP* reporter.) I) Cross section of the calyx in the adult brain, showing areas of arborisations of each of the four clonal units. (Data by Nobuaki Karl Tanaka. MARCM clone with UAS-*GFP* reporter.) J: Scheme of the four-fold clonal units in the MB.

Note on the name of the lobes: The names of the lobes have been changed drastically during the last few years of the last century. The terms of the α and β lobes originated from the study of the bee brain[60] to refer to the vertical and medial lobes. The γ lobe derived from the study of sphinx moth.[61] These terms are adopted to describe the fly MB.[2,62] Because of the apparent structural similarity, vertical and medial lobes in the larval MB had also been called as larval α and β lobes.[36]

Analysis of clones and GAL4 enhancer-trap strains revealed a characteristic subdivision of the α lobe and defined it as the α' lobe, but failed to recognise the corresponding subdivision in the β lobe.[36] The latter subdivision was identified by the comparison of labelling pattern of various antibodies and named as the β' lobe.[3] Until this period, it was not known that the neurons innervating the γ lobe have no vertical branches. Though such unbranched neurons had been observed in Golgi impregnated samples, the non-existence of the branch could not be determined conclusively because Golgi labelling may not always label all the branches of a neuron.

Finally, systematic flippase-mediated single-cell analyses revealed that the neurons contributing to the γ lobe, α'/β' lobes and α/β lobes are generated in this order and that the vertical and medial lobes of the larval MB is contributed exclusively by the neurons that compose the adult γ lobe as a result of reorganization.[41] The larval vertical and medial lobes, therefore, have nothing to do with the neurons of the adult α/β lobes.

To avoid confusion, it is better not to use the term α/β lobes for the larval MB but to use the generic term vertical/medial lobes instead. Also, the adult vertical lobe should not generally be called the α lobe, as it actually consists of α and α' lobes each of which is likely to have rather different functions.

The vertical and medial lobes are sometimes called dorsal and horizontal lobes, respectively. In various insects, however, the vertical lobe does not project dorsally but anteriorly or anterodorsally. The medial lobe projects medially (towards the midline) in all insect species, but the inclination of the lobe may not always be horizontal. Thus, the combination of "vertical" and "medial" seems more appropriate when considering cross-species compatibility. A-G, J reproduced with permission of the Company of Biologists.

trans-*Recombination Systems*

One of the classic methods for analysing lineage-associated cells is to induce somatic recombination by irradiating the animals with X ray or γ ray. Recombined cells can be identified by putting a marker gene in one of the chromosomes. As a more controllable and easy-to-use approach, FRT was put into the chromosome to induce flippase-dependent *trans*-recombination.[34] The lack of convenient reporter systems for detecting the neurons that experienced recombination has made it difficult to apply this technique for brain research. The mosaic analysis with a repressible cell marker (MARCM) system solved this problem.[39] The MARCM system features GAL80, which works antagonistically to GAL4 (Fig. 2E). GAL80 suppresses expression of the UAS-linked reporter gene even in the presence of GAL4. Flippase-induced somatic recombination between the FRT sequences removes *GAL80* gene in one of the daughter cells. UAS-linked reporter/effecter genes will be expressed specifically in this cell and its progeny.

An advantage of the MARCM system is that it can be combined with the somatic recombination analysis of recessive mutations, so that only the cells that are homozygous for the mutation can be visualised. This has been proven as highly effective tool for studying cell-autonomous roles of various genes during development.

Clonal Unit Architecture in the Adult Brain

Clonal Units in the Mushroom Body

The correlation between cell lineage and adult neural circuits was first identified in the MB. Although most neuroblasts proliferate at two separated periods in *Drosophila*, there are five neuroblasts that proliferate continuously throughout neurogenesis.[7] By administrating bromodeoxyuridine (BrdU) to larvae just after hatching, it is possible to label the nuclei of these proliferating neuroblasts and their progeny. One neuroblast lies in the anteriorlateral area of the larval brain and its progeny is distributed in the lateral side of the AL in the adult. The other four neuroblasts lie in the posterior dorsal area of the larval brain and their progeny are found lying above the MB calyx. Though BrdU can visualise only the nuclei of the labelled cells, their positions on the calyx strongly suggested that they are the MB Kenyon cells.

A more direct evidence came later with the advanced genetic analysis using flippase-mediated *cis*- or *trans*-recombination analyses, which enabled visualisation of neurites of the clonally related cells.[36,39] When clones are labelled early during development and visualised in a late larval stage, a single neuroblast, a few large GMCs and many small neurons are labelled (Fig. 3A-C). They innervate only within the MB neuropile. The cell bodies of the clonally related progeny remain in a tightly bound cluster in the adult brain, indicating that the cells do not migrate long distances from their place of origin. All the fibres deriving from this cluster innervate the MB, with no projection to other brain areas (Fig. 3D-F). Thus, these clones are indeed dedicated to the neural circuit of the MB.

There should be four different clonally-related populations each deriving from one of the four neuroblasts. Are they different from each other? The clusters of cell bodies are observed in four areas of the rind above the calyx and neurites from these clusters form four large bundles that run around the lower part of the calyx. The fibres from each cluster contribute to all the known components of the MB: the calyx, pedunculus and the α'/β', α/β and γ lobes. Thus, concerning the area of projection, the neurons of four clones are essentially identical.

The four-fold structure of the MB is further confirmed by the observation of GAL4 enhancer-trap strains. There are many GAL4 strains that label various subsets of the Kenyon cells, suggesting that the MB should consist of a heterogeneous population of neurons concerning their gene expression patterns.[36,40] These strains all label neurons in each of the four clusters, indicating that each clone essentially contains an identical repertoire of Kenyon cells. The four-fold pattern is most evident in the strains that label Kenyon cells innervating the α/β lobes, which are generated latest during development[41] (top panel of Fig. 3G). The four bundles of clonally related neurons are clearly labelled at the level of the calyx. The bundles deriving from the two medial clusters and two lateral clusters (1, 2 and 3, 4 in Fig. 3G, respectively) are fused in the middle level of the calyx. The two merged bundles further merge at the anterior end of the pedunculus. The neurites from each clonal cluster are intermingled completely in the lobe area. The four bundles are discernible but are less clear in the strains that label a variety of Kenyon cells (middle panel of Fig. 3G). The discrete pattern is more ambiguous in the strains that label neurons projecting only to the γ lobe, because their neurites run near the surface of the pedunculus (bottom panel of Fig. 3G).

There are, however, certain differences between the four clones concerning the types of information they receive. The MB receives olfactory signals from the antennal lobe, which is conveyed by the antennal lobe projection neurons (AL PNs). Many of them are uniglomerular, sending signals from one particular glomerulus of the AL to the MB (see Chapter by V Rodrigues and T Hummel). In larvae, terminals of these AL PNs form small glomerular structures in the calyx called microglomeruli[42,43] (see also Chapter by R Stocker). Their positions are reproducible among individuals, showing that olfactory information from particular glomeruli in the larval AL is transmitted to distinct subregions of the calyx. The arborisations of the Kenyon cells of each clone occupy different, but partially overlapping, areas of the calyx (Fig. 3H).[42] Thus, each clone should receive a different repertoire of olfactory information.

Because of the much larger number of AL PNs and the number of glomeruli in the adult AL, there are numerous very small microglomeruli in the calyx of the adult MB, making their mapping more complex (see Chapter by P Laissue and L Vosshall). Nevertheless, AL PNs from particular AL glomerulus terminate in specific concentric zones in the calyx.[4] The Kenyon cells of each clone again arborise in distinct areas of the calyx (Fig. 3I),[4,44] suggesting that there may also be differences in the repertoire of olfactory information each clone would receive. For example, the two "outer" clones (1 and 4 in Fig. 3I) may have fewer interaction with the projection neurons that terminate in the central area of the calyx than do the two "inner" clones (2 and 3 of Fig. 3I).

Observations in the MB suggest that there are clonally-related unit structures in the adult brain. Progeny of a single neuroblast may contain a functionally heterogeneous population of neurons. Yet, they all innervate only a limited area of the brain and form a distinct neural circuit structure. There are four such clonal units in the *Drosophila* MB, which are essentially identical regarding their morphology and biochemical diversity but slightly different in the projection pattern in their input areas (Fig. 3J).

Clonal Unit Architecture in the Central Complex

Clonal unit is not a unique feature of the MB. They are also observed in the central complex, the neuropile that lies at the centre of the cerebrum[2,4,5] and is supposed to play important roles in motor coordination control, visual memory, etc.[46-48] The structure of the central complex is much more complex than the MB (Fig. 4A). It consists of four major components, the ellipsoid body (eb), fan-shaped body (fb), protocerebral bridge (pb) and noduli (no).[45] Whereas the cell bodies of the MB Kenyon cells are all confined in a small area just around the MB calyx, those that contribute to the central complex are distributed in various parts of the brain. Nevertheless, lineage-dependent cell labelling experiments revealed that several clones contribute specifically to the central complex, each forming distinct building units of its neural circuits.

The ellipsoid body is a round structure that forms the anteriormost part of the central complex. There is a pair of clonal units with their cell bodies in the anterior brain above the aimpr area of the cerebrum, dorsolateral to the AL (EB-A1, Fig. 4A,B). A bundle of neurites projects beneath the medial lobe of the MB and forms the primary arborisation in the vmpr part of the cerebrum, forming the structure called the lateral triangle (ltr). From the ltr, some fibres project dorsally to reach the asmpr and aimpr and others project to the ellipsoid body from its central hole to form the ring neurons of this neuropile.

The fan-shaped body consists of an array of radial projections and tangential neurons that arborise at its various dorsoventral levels. One of the clonal units that form these tangential components have the cell body cluster in the dorsolateral area of the cerebrum, posterior to the LH (FB-DL1, Fig. 4A,C). The neurons form primary arborisations near the dorsal surface of the cerebrum above the LH and secondary arborisations in the msmpr and mslpr. The fibre bundle bifurcates, enters the fan-shaped body from its anterior side at two levels (Fig. 4C) and forms extensive branches that span tangentially. There are also other clonal units that form tangential arborisations in different levels of the fan-shaped body (not shown here).

The radial component of the fan-shaped body is formed by four clonal units per hemisphere (FB-P1-4, Fig. 4A,D). A row of eight cell body clusters lies in the posterior brain right behind the fan-shaped body, flanked by the calyces of the MB. The neurites form primary arborisation in the protocerebral bridge and enter the inferior part of the fan-shaped body from its posterior side. They form two bundles that run radially in the fan-shaped body and terminate in the nodulus of the contralateral hemisphere.

The protocerebral bridge is divided into eight sections per hemisphere. Similarly, the radial component of the fan-shaped body is organized in eight radial structures called the staves.[2,45]

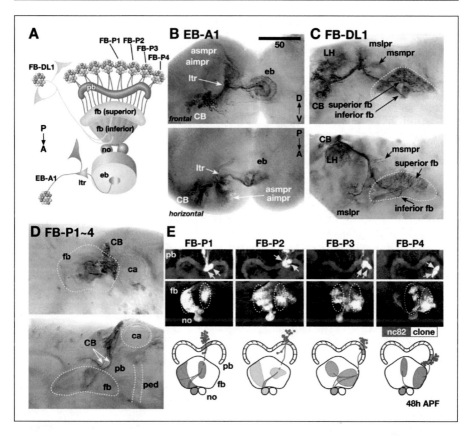

Figure 4. Clonal units in the central complex. A) Scheme of the central complex and three major types of clonally related components. There are also several other clonal units that contribute to the central complex. *pb*: protocerebral bridge, *fb*: fan-shaped body, *no*: nodulus, *eb*: ellipsoid body, *ltr*: lateral triangle. B-D) Examples of clonal units contributing to the central complex. See legend to Figure 1 for neuropile regions. FLP-out-GAL4 clones visualised with UAS-*tau* reporter in the adult brain. Top and bottom photographs of each figure show the montage of optical sections of the same clone in frontal and horizontal view, respectively. Clonal units: EB-A1 (ellipsoid body-anterior 1, B), FB-DL1 (fan-shaped body dorsolateral 1, C) and FB-P1-4 (fan-shaped body posterior 1-4, D). E) Arborisation areas of the four FB-P clonal units (Data by Mariko Kamiya). Confocal sections at the level of the protocerebral bridge (top panel), fan-shaped body and nodulus (middle panel) and the schema of the projection pattern (bottom panel). (MARCM clone with UAS-*GFP* reporter in the mid pupal brain 48 h after puparium formation, when the neuropile structure is already essentially the same as in the adult.)

Neurites of each FB-P clonal unit arborise in two sections of the protocerebral bridge (Fig. 4E, top panel) and contribute to two staves of the fan-shaped body (Fig. 4D, bottom panel). Collateral fibres deriving from these staves arborise in two areas of the fan-shaped body, one in the ipsilateral and the other in the contralateral side (Fig. 4E, middle panel). Whereas the arborisation of each clonal unit is segregated in the protocerebral bridge, there is a significantly overlap between their arborisations in the fan-shaped body. In the nodulus, fibres of all the four clonal units converge and arborise in the entire area of its neuropile (Fig. 4E, bottom panel).

Clonal Unit Architecture in Other Brain Areas

Compared to the MB and the central complex, borders between neural circuits in the rest of the central brain are much more obscure. Nevertheless, clonally related neurons innervate only limited areas of these neuropiles and form distinct unit structures.

Projection neurons from the antennal lobe innervate the MB calyx, the LH and several other areas of the brain.[13,14] GAL4 enhancer-trap strains such as GH146, NP225 and NP5288 label many of these neurons.[4,49,50] The cell bodies of these neurons form at least four clusters around the AL. The anterior dorsal cluster (AL-DA1, Fig. 5A) and a lateral cluster (AL-L1, not shown here) consists of the neurons that innervate via the inner antennocerebral tract (iACT). The cell cluster that lies ventral to the AL (AL-V1, not shown here) consists of the neurons of the middle ACT (mACT) pathway. There is yet another clone in the lateral area of the AL, which consists of the neurons that do not seem to be labelled in these GAL4 strains (AL-L2, Fig. 5B). Neurons of this clonal unit project not only to the MB and calyx but also to the SOG and the plpr.

In the MB, neurons other than the Kenyon cells also innervate its neuropile. An example of such clonal unit, MB-A1 (Fig. 5C), has the cell bodies in the anterior brain just in front of the MB vertical lobe.[10] Neurons of this clone mainly innervate the distal area of the medial lobe and project also to the neuropiles other than the MB in the aimpr and vmpr areas.

Neurons in the LH, which receives olfactory information from the AL like the MB Kenyon cells, are also organized in a clonally related manner. Several clonal units contribute to the neuropile of the LH. Their cell bodies form clusters in the LCBR. Some clones (e.g., LH-1, Fig. 5D) consist of local neurons that arborise only in the LH. The neurites of other clones (e.g., LH-2 and 3, Fig. 5E,F) arborise in the LH and project further to other areas of the protocerebral neuropiles. Depending on the clonal units, the neurites project to the LH either from inside (LH-2,3) or from outside (LH-1).

The superior lateral and superior medial protocerebrum occupies the dorsalmost area of the cerebrum. Because neural connections between these neuropiles and the neuropiles of the sensory and motor pathways are still essentially unknown, the function of the neural circuits in these areas are yet to be determined. These neuropiles are also contributed by many clonal units. Short of the knowledge of determining neural structure in these areas, these clonal units are tentatively named according to the neuropile region (Fig. 1H-N) in which they arborise most extensively. Some clonal units, e.g., PSLPR-1 and MSLPR-1 (Fig. 5G,H), arborise only in a small region of the neuropile. They tend to have simple structures, with a single bundle of neurites and arborisation in one or only a few areas. Other clones, like MSLPR-2 and MSMPR-1 (Fig. 5I,J), arborise in multiple areas. The structure of these clonal units are more complex, with bifurcation or trifurcation of neurite bundles and extensive projections that span a long distance in the brain.

The ventrolateral part of the cerebrum (vlpr and plpr) is occupied by the neuropiles that extensively receive axons of the visual projection neurons, which connect the optic lobe and the central brain.[2,5] These areas are also formed by various clonal units, whose cell bodies lie in the LCBR or in the anterior lateral area of the cerebrum. Some clonal units form circuits that connect the corresponding neuropiles of both hemispheres (e.g., VLPR-1, Fig. 5K), whereas others connect a variety of neuropile areas of the cerebrum (e.g., VLPR-2, Fig. 5L).

Formation of the Clonal Units During Development

The observations presented above suggest that a significant portion of the adult brain is composed in a cell lineage-dependent manner (Fig. 2B). Though the progeny of a single neuroblast are not as tightly packed as in the larval brain, they still form a cluster. Neurites deriving from this cluster form tight bundles and innervate distinct areas of the brain.

How, then, is such clonal unit architecture in the adult brain composed during neurogenesis? When the clones are visualised in late larval or early pupal brains, the progeny of a neuroblast form a tightly packed cluster, which sends a bundle of neurites towards the neuropile (Fig. 6A,B). The bundle either projects to a single target or bifurcates when it enters the neuropile to innervate different areas of the brain.[51] The formation of the adult clonal units should depend on this

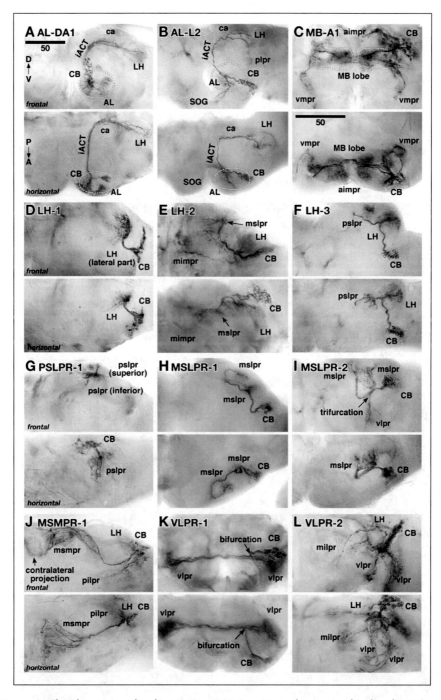

Figure 5. Clonal units in other brain areas. FLP-out-GAL4 clones visualised with UAS-*tau* reporter. Top and bottom photographs of each figure (A-L) show the montage of frontal and horizontal optical sections of the same sample, respectively. See legend to Figure 1 for neuropile regions.

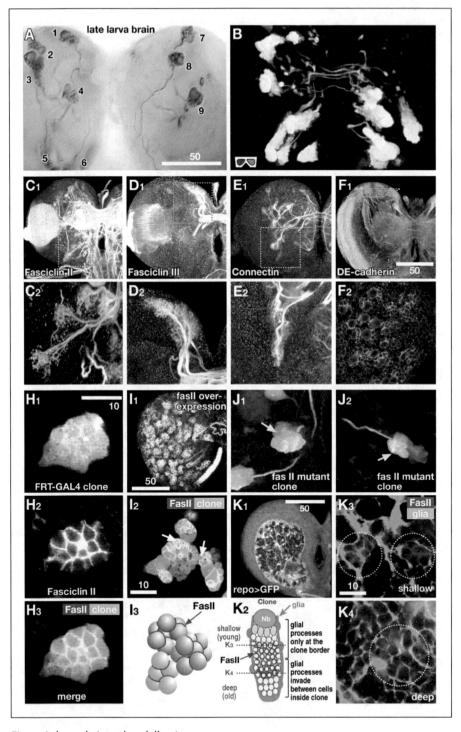

Figure 6, legend viewed on following page.

Figure 6, viewed on previous page. Formation of clonal units in the larval brain. A, B) Clonal units in late larvae. FLP-out-GAL4 clones visualised with UAS-*tau* (A, montage of optical sections) and UAS-*GFP* (B, 3D-stereograph of confocal sections). C-F) Distribution of cell-adhesion molecules in the larval brain visualised with antibodies. Overall brain (top panel) and blow-up view (bottom panel) showing the area indicated with dashed squares in the top panel. Clonal-unit dependent distribution of Fasciclin II (FasII, C), Fasciclin III (D) and Connectin (E) and pan-clonal distribution of DE-cadherin (F). H) Distribution of FasII visualised with anti-FasII antibody in the cluster of clonal cell bodies. I) Over-expression of FasII in all the neurons (using elav-*GAL4C155* driver, I1) and in the MARCM clones (I2). J) Effect of the homozygous mutation of FasII in the MARCM clones. Two examples are shown. K) Distribution of FasII (visualised with anti-FasII antibody) and glial processes (visualised with UAS-*GFP* driven with glia-specific repo-GAL4 driver).

clonal cluster formation in larvae. Because formation of the lineage-dependent structure in the larval brain is comprehensively described in the Chapter by V Hartenstein et al, here we discuss this issue only briefly.

One of the candidate mechanisms that promote binding of the clonally related cell bodies and neurites depends on homophilic cell adhesion molecules (CAMs). If such CAMs are expressed in the clonally related neurons, they would facilitate adhesion of the cells and fibre bundles.[51-53]

According to their expression patterns, the homophilic CAMs can be classified into two types. The first type is expressed only in a small subset of the clones. This includes Fasciclin II (Fas II), Fasciclin III (Fas III) and Connectin (Fig. 6C-E). Interestingly, whereas the expression patterns of these CAMs are associated with the clonal units in the developing brain, they are not related with the clonal units in the adult. This suggests that intra-clonal cell-cell adhesion would be mediated by these CAMs during the formation of certain clones.

The other group is expressed in most of the developing clonal units: this category includes CAMs like DE-cadherin (DE-cad) and Neurotactin (Fig. 6F). The role of such pan-clonal CAMs during development has been studied using the ectopic expression of the dominant negative form of DE-cad, which affected the organisation of the developing clonal clusters.[54] Although the observed abnormality was not severe, the function of DE-cad at least seems to be involved in the correct formation of the clonal architecture.

The role of the clone-specific CAMs, on the other hand, is not yet clear. When the distribution of one such CAM, Fas II, is visualised together with the clonal cluster, the protein is observed only on the cell surface that is flanked by other siblings in the same clone but not on the outer surface of the cell body cluster (Fig. 6H). To determine whether Fas II is concentrated because of the homophilic interaction with the same molecule of the neighbouring cells, we over-expressed FasII so that cells in the neighbouring clones express the same protein. Even in this case, FasII is concentrated only along the cell border within each clone but not along the cell border between clones (Fig. 6I2, I3). Ectopic expression of FasII in all the neurons, which should negate the clone-specific role of this molecule, affect neither the organised distribution of the clonal cell clusters nor the projection patterns of neurites (Fig. 6I1). Moreover, the formation of the clonal cell cluster and neurite bundles is not disturbed even when the function of FasII is removed by inducing *fasII* mutant clones using the MARCM system (Fig. 6J). Thus, removal of just one clone-specific CAM does not affect the formation and maintenance of the clonal architecture in the larval brain. It is possible that pan-clonal and clone-specific CAMs might function cooperatively to facilitate the clone-specific cell-cell adhesion.

Another factor that would be important for the organisation of the clonal unit is the cell body glial cells, which send processes between neural cell bodies.[12] The region of the rind near the surface of the larval brain is characterised by the glial processes that form large nest-like holes (Fig. 6K1).[55] Because each glial nest houses a neuroblast and its progeny, the surface of the clonal cluster is flanked by the glial sheath. This organisation explains why FasII is accumulated only in the intraclonal border of the cell bodies (Fig. 6K3). Because glial cells do not express FasII, the glial sheath physically separates the cells of the FasII-expressing clones even when they are flanked with each other.

In the deeper level of the rind, glial processes invade borders between neural cell bodies of the clones. Though FasII is still distributed along the intraclonal cell border, neighbouring cell bodies are separated by the invaded glial processes (Fig. 6K4). In the adult, all the neural cell body in the rind are each surrounded by extensive glial processes (Fig. 1F, G). Thus, the glial nest seems to be a transiently structure formed due to the time required for the extension of glial processes during larval neurogenesis. Although glial cells continue invading all the space between neural cell bodies, a temporal delay is inevitable between the period when neurons are newly formed by the GMC and the time when glial cells outside of the clonal cluster send processes between them (Fig. 6K2). This delay results in the glial nest architecture in the larval brain. Clone-specific CAMs may stabilise the clustering of sibling neurons during this time lag. Since the cell clusters are buttressed by the sheath of the glial nest and because pan-clonal CAMs may function redundantly, over-expression or lack of a particular clone-specific CAM would not lead to significantly abnormal phenotypes.

Functional Importance of the Clonal Units

Because many areas of the brain neuropile are formed by the combination of clonal units, they seem to be the fundamental building blocks of the adult fly neural circuits. There would be several advantages by organising the brain in such a clone dependent manner. Unlike in the simple nervous system of early embryos, neural fibres in the postembryonic brain must find their paths through the three-dimensional space filled with tangled fibres of other neurons. If each neuron differentiates and sends its neurite independently, a large variety of attracting and repulsive signals would be required for providing positional cues for these neurons (Fig. 7A1).[56] Because neural fibres innervating different targets would criss-cross with each other, systems for avoiding unnecessary cross-talk between these signals would be inevitable. If neurons of the same cluster, on the other hand, form fascicles to project to only distinct areas of the brain, the guidance system for the follower neurons should be much simpler (Fig. 7A2). Path finding of individual neurons will be required only in the area near the target. Projection towards an additional target is a matter of locating the branching point in the one-dimensional space along the neurite bundle. Even in such clones, the first neuron (the so called pioneer neuron) has to extend its fibre without the help of a pre-exiting fascicle. As this occurs in relatively early embryos, when the brain neuropile is still simpler and the distance between the cell body and the target is much shorter than in the adult, path finding would be relatively easy.

Although flippase-mediated labelling visualises clonal units so clearly, few molecular markers such as antibodies and enhancer-trap strains label neurons of a single clonal unit. Rather, they tend to label small subsets of neurons scattered in many clonal units. This suggests that, although neurons of each clonal unit are relatively homogeneous regarding their overall projection patterns, they are rather heterogeneous concerning properties like gene expression patterns. They are also heterogeneous in the precise arborisations within the target areas. These suggest that a single clonal unit would be a versatile functional unit in which a variety of complicated computation is possible. Organising the brain by the composition of such units might have been an economical way for developing complicated neural circuits during evolution. Just like duplication and subsequent modification of genes added new functions to the genome, addition of new clonal units by the formation of additional neuroblasts might be a convenient way of incremental evolution of the brain (Fig. 7B). The loss of certain clonal units might also have occurred during evolution. Considering that there are several clonal units contributing overlappingly to the same circuit module of the brain (discussed later), such loss of clonal units may not have jeopardised the architecture and function of the brain.

Whereas some clonal units consist of several hundreds of neurons, some have less than 50 neurons. Such significant differences in cell number may affect the computational capacity of the circuits formed by that clonal unit. Because different insect species rely on very different sensory signals depending on their habitats and life styles, computational requirements for the evolutionary comparable clonal units might vary. Not only duplication or removal of clonal units but also the change in the cell numbers of clones might have been important during evolution. Though

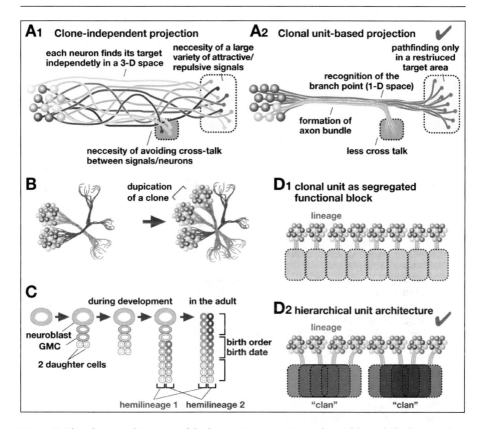

Figure 7. Clonal unit architecture of the brain. A) Comparison of possible path-finding mechanisms between clone-independent (left) and clone-dependent (right) organisation of the brain. B) Hypothetical scheme of incremental complication of neural circuits. C) Possible factors that affect the diversity of neurons within each clone. D) Scheme of the arborisation area of each clonal unit. Each clone innervates segregated areas of the neuropile (D1), or, Several clones innervate highly overlapping areas to form functional modules of the brain (D2).

visualisation of the clonal units in the adult brain is currently possible only in *Drosophila*, comparative study of clonal units across insect taxa in the future would provide important insights on the functional composition of the brain.

As for the heterogeneity within each clonal unit, there would be two candidate control factors (Fig. 7C). The first factor is the order and timing of cell generation. During embryonic development, neuroblasts change their gene expression pattern drastically and neurons that are made at each time point are characteristically affected by this.[19,57] In the postembryonic stages, expression patterns of the neuroblasts do not seem to change so quickly. Nevertheless, specific projection patterns of the adult neurons in the target area, such as the arborisation of AL-PNs in the AL and the LH and that of the MB Kenyon cells in the lobes, are dependent on the birth date of each neuron during larval stage.[41,49] A BTB zinc-finger protein gene has been identified that governs neuronal temporal identity during postembryonic fly brain development.[58] Expression levels of this molecule in the clonal neurons are reduced gradually depending on their birth timing. Temporal gradient in the activity of such genes may specify cell fate in an extended neuronal lineage.

Other factors would control the differences between the two sibling neurons made by each of the GMCs. Proteins such as Numb are distributed unevenly between the two daughter cells, activating the Notch signalling pathway in only one of them. This difference between sibling cells of the olfactory sensory neurons made by the same precursor causes clustering of projection targets in the AL.[59] Similar differences between sister cells, each of which comprises a "hemilineage", may occur within the clonal units of the brain (Fig. 7C).

The concept of the adult brain made by the building blocks of clonal units may give the impression that each clone occupies specific and discrete areas of the brain neuropile (Fig. 7D1). Indeed, 3D reconstruction of clonal units yields images of clonally related neuronal fibres that appear to fill particular areas of the brain. This, however, might be a too simplistic view. Because the diameter of neural fibres is much smaller than the resolution of the optical microscopes, dense arborisation is visualized as a solid structure even when only a fraction of the volume is occupied by the visualised fibres. Volume- and surface-rendering algorithms of the 3D reconstruction software further remove fine detail of the visualised fibres, oversimplifying the projection pattern in the area. For the neurons of each clonal unit to communicate with neurons of other units, their arborisations have to be spatially colocalised and therefore intermingled. Thus, clonal units should in principle contribute to significantly overlapping areas of the brain (Fig. 7D2). Interestingly, the degree of overlap appears to be larger in the arborisation areas that are distal from the cell body clusters. Both in the MB and FB-P clones, arborisations of each clone occupy distinct areas in the calyx and protocerebral bridge but overlap completely in the lobes and nodulli (Figs. 3J,4E).

The degree of overlap between specific sets of clonal units is much larger than the overlap with the rest of the clones. In another word, several clonal units contribute together to form distinct neural circuit units, to which other clones contribute only marginally. In these cases, the neural circuit formed by each clonal unit may be too small and simple to represent an independent functional unit. The neural circuits in the brain are therefore organised in a hierarchical manner. Neurons deriving from several cell lineages form a "clan", which together contribute to the formation of a functional module of the brain circuit. The four clonal units of the MB, several clonal units around the AL that all arborise in the AL and form the complete set of ACT pathways, clones in the anterior and posterior brain that together compose the central complex neuropile, are examples of such clans. The clan might therefore be as important as lineage for understanding the functional dynamics of the brain, just like a clan of people, who belong to a number of tightly-associated lineages, behaved as a functional group in the dynamics of the ancient human society (Fig. 7D2).

Conclusion

Complicated neural circuits in the brain are composed by the combination of relatively simple clonal units. A group of clonal units together form a functional module of the brain. Developmental mechanisms that form such lineage- and clan-dependent structures are not yet fully understood. Guidance molecules and interactions between neurites of the same clone and between those of the neighbouring clones would play important roles in this process. More detailed analysis of the arborisation patterns and gene expression patterns of the neurons of each clonal unit would be required. Analysis of temporal aspects, not only about the order of neuron formation within each clone but also about the timing of proliferation and neurite extension among clones of the same clan, would also further our understanding about the process of the neural circuit formation.

Acknowledgements

We are grateful to Kazumi Suzuki and Mariko Kamiya for the preparation of images of the clonal units, Nobuaki Karl Tanaka for the unpublished data of the arborisation pattern of the clonal units in the adult calyx and Liria Masuda-Nakagawa for the reproduction of images in the larval calyx. This work is supported by the grants of the Precursory Research for Embryonic Science and Technology and the Institute for Bioinformatics Research and Development from Japan Science and Technology Agency to KI and TA and the Grant-in-Aid for Scientific Research from the Ministry of Education, Culture, Sports, Science and Technology of Japan to KI.

References

1. Power ME. The brain of Drosophila. J Morph 1943; 72:517-559.
2. Strausfeld NJ. Atlas of an Insect Brain. Berlin, Heidelberg, New York, Tokyo: Springer-Verlag, 1976.

3. Crittenden JR, Skoulakis EM, Han KA et al. Tripartite mushroom body architecture revealed by antigenic markers. Learn Mem 1998; 5:38-51.
4. Tanaka NK, Awasaki T, Shimada T et al. Integration of chemosensory pathways in the Drosophila second-order olfactory centers. Curr Biol 2004; 14:449-457.
5. Otsuna H, Ito K. Systematic analysis of the visual projection neurons of Drosophila melanogaster I. Lobula-specific pathways. J Comp Neurol 2006; 497:928-958.
6. Truman JW, Bate M. Spatial and temporal patterns of neurogenesis in the central nervous system of Drosophila melanogaster. Dev Biol 1988; 125:145-157.
7. Ito K, Hotta Y. Proliferation pattern of postembryonic neuroblasts in the brain of Drosophila melanogaster. Dev Biol 1992; 149:134-148.
8. Fischbach KF, Dittrich APM. The optic lobe of Drosophila melanogaster I. A golgi analysis of wild-type structure. Cell Tissue Res 1989; 258:441-475.
9. Bausenwein B, Dittrich APM, Fischbach KF. The optic lobe of Drosophila melanogaster II. Sorting of retinotopic pathways in the medulla. Cell Tissue Res 1992; 267:17-28.
10. Ito K, Suzuki K, Estes P et al. The organization of extrinsic neurons and their implications in the functional roles of the mushroom bodies in Drosophila melanogaster Meigen. Learn Mem 1998; 5:52-77.
11. Wagh DA, Rasse TM, Asan E et al. Bruchpilot, a protein with homology to ELKS/CAST, is required for structural integrity and function of synaptic active zones in Drosophila. Neuron 2006; 49:833-844.
12. Ito K, Urban J, Technau GM. Distribution, classification and development of Drosophila glial cells in the late embryonic and early larval ventral nerve cord. Roux's Arch Dev Biol 1995; 204:284-307.
13. Stocker RF, Lienhard MC, Borst A et al. Neuronal architecture of the antennal lobe in Drosophila melanogaster. Cell Tissue Res 1990; 262:9-34.
14. Stocker RF. The organization of the chemosensory system in Drosophila melanogaster: a review. Cell Tissue Res 1994; 275:3-26.
15. Kamikouchi A, Shimada T, Ito K. Comprehensive classification of the auditory sensory projections in the brain of the fruit fly Drosophila melanogaster. J Comp Neurol 2006; 499:317-356.
16. Hofbauer A, Campos-Ortega JA. Proliferation pattern and early differentiation of the optic lobes in Drosophila melanogaster. Roux's Arch Dev Biol 1990; 198:264-274.
17. Prokop A, Technau GM. The origin of postembryonic neuroblasts in the ventral nerve cord of Drosophila melanogaster. Development 1991; 111:79-88.
18. Urbach R, Schnabel R, Technau GM. The pattern of neuroblast formation, mitotic domains and proneural gene expression during early brain development in Drosophila. Development 2003; 130:3589-3606.
19. Urbach R, Technau GM. Molecular markers for identified neuroblasts in the developing brain of Drosophila. Development 2003; 130:3621-3637.
20. Technau GM, Campos-Ortega JA. Fate-mapping in wild-type Drosophila melanogaster. II. Injections of horseradish peroxidase in cells of the early gatrula stage. Roux's Arch Dev Biol 1985; 194:196-212.
21. Bossing T, Technau GM. The fate of the CNS midline progenitors in Drosophila as revealed by a new method for single cell labelling. Development 1994; 120:1895-1906.
22. Bossing T, Udolph G, Doe CQ et al. The embryonic central nervous system lineages of Drosophila melanogaster. I. Neuroblast lineages derived from the ventral half of the neuroectoderm. Dev Biol 1996; 179:41-64.
23. Schmidt H, Rickert C, Bossing T et al. The embryonic central nervous system lineages of Drosophila melanogaster II. Neuroblast lineages derived from the dorsal part of the neuroectoderm. Dev Biol 1997; 189:186-204.
24. Schmid A, Chiba A, Doe CQ. Clonal analysis of Drosophila embryonic neuroblasts: neural cell types, axon projections and muscle targets. Development 1999; 126:4653-4689.
25. Technau GM. Lineage analysis of transplanted individual cells in embryos of Drosophila melanogaster I. The method. Roux's Arch Dev Biol 1986; 195:389-398.
26. Technau GM, Campos-Ortega JA. Lineage analysis of transplanted individual cells in embryos of Drosophila melanogaster II. Commitment and proliferative capabilities of neural and epidermal cell progenitors. Roux's Arch Dev Biol 1986; 195:445-454.
27. Technau GM, Campos-Ortega JA. Lineage analysis of transplanted individual cells in embryos of Drosophila melanogaster III. Commitment and proliferative capabilities of pole cells and midgut progenitors. Roux's Arch Dev Biol 1986; 195:489-498.
28. Prokop A, Technau GM. Early tagma-specific commitment of Drosophila CNS progenitor NB1-1. Development 1994; 120:2567-2578.
29. Fischer JA, Giniger E, Maniatis T et al. GAL4 activates transcription in Drosophila. Nature 1988; 332:853-856.
30. Brand AH, Perrimon N. Targeted gene expression as a means of altering cell fates and generating dominant phenotypes. Development 1993; 118:401-415.
31. Brand AH, Dormand EL. The GAL4 system as a tool for unravelling the mysteries of the Drosophila nervous system. Curr Opin Neurobiol 1995; 5:572-578.

32. Golic KG, Lindquist S. The FLP recombinase of yeast catalyzes site-specific recombination in the Drosophila genome. Cell 1989; 59:499-509.
33. Dang DT, Perrimon N. Use of a yeast site-specific recombinase to generate embryonic mosaics in Drosophila. Dev Genet 1992; 13:367-375.
34. Xu T, Rubin GM. Analysis of genetic mosaics in developing and adult Drosophila tissues. Development 1993; 117:1223-1237.
35. Struhl G, Basler K. Organizing activity of wingless protein in Drosophila. Cell 1993; 72:527-540.
36. Ito K, Awano W, Suzuki K et al. The Drosophila mushroom body is a quadruple structure of clonal units each of which contains a virtually identical set of neurones and glial cells. Development 1997; 124:761-771.
37. Basler K, Struhl G. Compartment boundaries and the control of Drosophila limb pattern by hedgehog protein. Nature 1994; 368:208-214.
38. Wong AM, Wang JW, Axel R. Spatial representation of the glomerular map in the Drosophila protocerebrum. Cell 2002; 109:229-241.
39. Lee T, Luo L. Mosaic analysis with a repressible cell marker for studies of gene function in neuronal morphogenesis. Neuron 1999; 22:451-461.
40. Yang MY, Armstrong JD, Vilinsky I et al. Subdivision of the Drosophila mushroom bodies by enhancer-trap expression patterns. Neuron 1995; 15:45-54.
41. Lee T, Lee A, Luo L. Development of the Drosophila mushroom bodies: sequential generation of three distinct types of neurons from a neuroblast. Development 1999; 126:4065-4076.
42. Masuda-Nakagawa LM, Tanaka NK, O'Kane CJ. Stereotypic and random patterns of connectivity in the larval mushroom body calyx of Drosophila. Proc Natl Acad Sci USA 2005; 102:19027-19032.
43. Ramaekers A, Magnenat E, Marin EC et al. Glomerular maps without cellular redundancy at successive levels of the Drosophila larval olfactory circuit. Curr Biol 2005; 15:982-992.
44. Zhu S, Chiang AS, Lee T. Development of the Drosophila mushroom bodies: elaboration, remodeling and spatial organization of dendrites in the calyx. Development 2003; 130:2603-2610.
45. Hanesch U, Fischbach KF, Heisenberg M. Neuronal architecture of the central complex in Drosophila melanogaster. Cell Tissue Res 1989; 257:343-366.
46. Strauss R, Heisenberg M. A higher control center of locomotor behavior in the Drosophila brain. J Neurosci 1993; 13:1852-1861.
47. Strauss R. The central complex and the genetic dissection of locomotor behaviour. Curr Opin Neurobiol 2002; 12:633-638.
48. Liu G, Seiler H, Wen A et al. Distinct memory traces for two visual features in the Drosophila brain. Nature 2006; 439:551-556.
49. Jefferis GS, Marin EC, Stocker RF et al. Target neuron prespecification in the olfactory map of Drosophila. Nature 2001; 414:204-208.
50. Marin EC, Jefferis GS, Komiyama T et al. Representation of the glomerular olfactory map in the Drosophila brain. Cell 2002; 109:243-255.
51. Pereanu W, Hartenstein V. Neural lineages of the Drosophila brain: a three-dimensional digital atlas of the pattern of lineage location and projection at the late larval stage. J Neurosci 2006; 26:5534-5553.
52. Akong K, McCartney BM, Peifer M. Drosophila APC2 and APC1 have overlapping roles in the larval brain despite their distinct intracellular localizations. Dev Biol 2002; 250:71-90.
53. Nassif C, Noveen A, Hartenstein V. Early development of the Drosophila brain: III. The pattern of neuropile founder tracts during the larval period. J Comp Neurol 2003; 455:417-434.
54. Dumstrei K, Wang F, Hartenstein V. Role of DE-cadherin in neuroblast proliferation, neural morphogenesis and axon tract formation in Drosophila larval brain development. J Neurosci 2003; 23:3325-3335.
55. Pereanu W, Shy D, Hartenstein V. Morphogenesis and proliferation of the larval brain glia in Drosophila. Dev Biol 2005; 283:191-203.
56. Tessier-Lavigne M, Goodman CS. The molecular biology of axon guidance. Science 1996; 274:1123-1133.
57. Isshiki T, Pearson B, Holbrook S et al. Drosophila neuroblasts sequentially express transcription factors which specify the temporal identity of their neuronal progeny. Cell 2001; 106:511-21.
58. Zhu S, Lin S, Kao CF et al. Gradients of the Drosophila Chinmo BTB-zinc finger protein govern neuronal temporal identity. Cell 2006; 127:409-422.
59. Endo K, Aoki T, Yoda Y et al. Notch signal organizes the Drosophila olfactory circuitry by diversifying the sensory neuronal lineages. Nat Neurosci 2007; 10:153-160.
60. Vowles D. The structure and connections of the corpora pedunculata in bees and ants. Q J Microsc Sci 1955; 96:239-255.
61. Pearson L. The corpora pedunculata of Sphinx ligustri L. and other Lepidoptera: an anatomical study. Philos Trans R Soc Lond B 1972; 259:477-516.
62. Heisenberg M. Mutants of brain structure and function: what is the significance of the mushroom bodies for behavior? Basic Life Sci 1980; 16:373-390.

INDEX